Shiatsu Uncovered

Ancient Wisdom for Modern Living

Mei Lin Zhang

Xspurts.com

A New Zealand Designed Product

Other Versions Available

Why limit yourself to just one format?

This book is now available in physical, digital, and audiobook options.

Choose the way you love to read and dive into the story today. You won't regret it!

Digital ISBN: 9781776968190
Physical ISBN: 9781776968183
Audio ISBN:

To obtain a different format of this book at a discounted price, please get in touch with us at:

http://isbn.xspurts.com/

Contents

Have Questions / Comments?

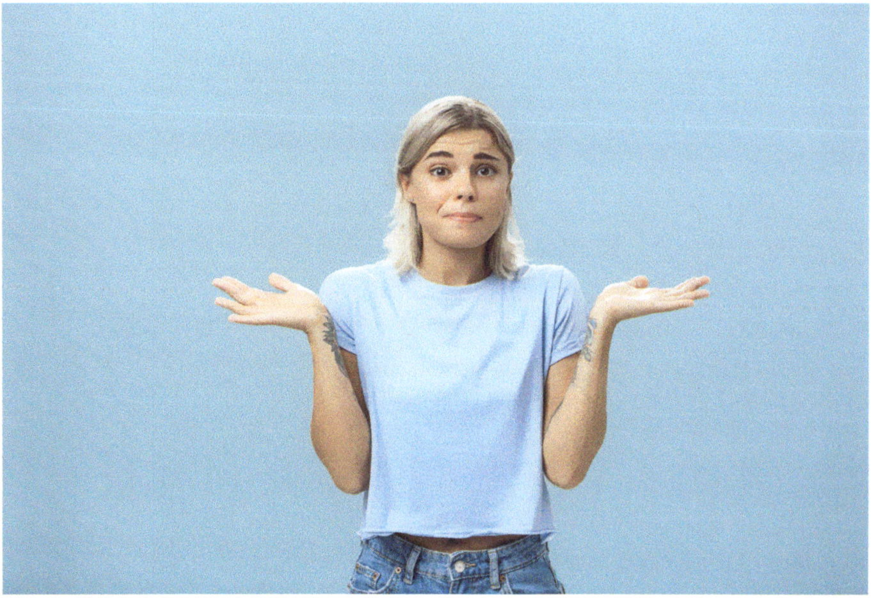

This book was designed to cover as much information as possible, but I know I have probably missed something, or some new amazing discovery has just come out.

If you notice something missing or have a question that I failed to answer, please get in touch and let me know. If I can, I will email you an answer and also update the book so others can also benefit from it.

Thanks For Being Awesome :)

Submit Your Questions / Comments At:

https://questions.xspurts.com

Get Free Stuff

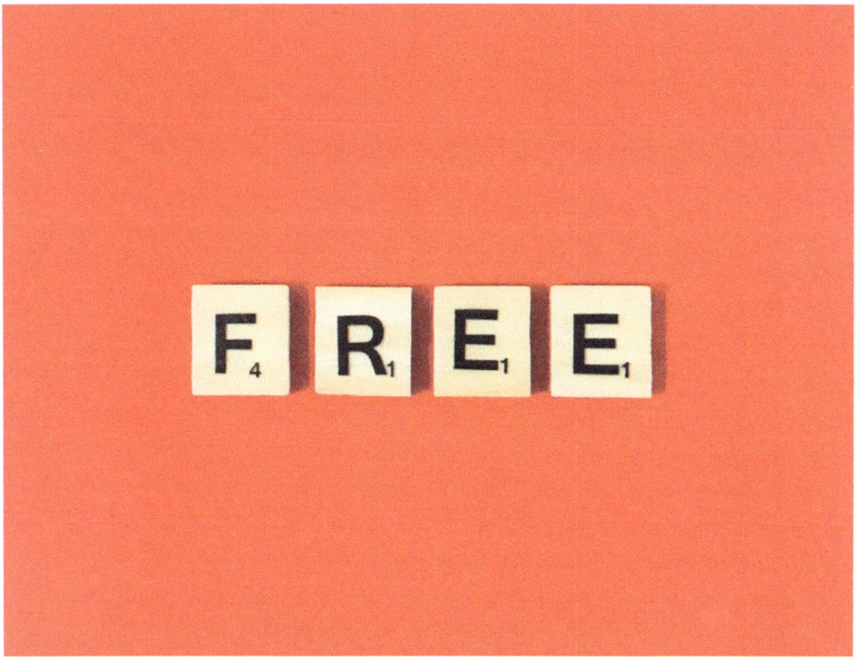

We love writing and have produced a huge number of books.

For being one of our amazing readers, we would love to offer you more books we have created, 100% free.

To claim this limited time special offer, simply go to the site below and enter your name and email address.

You will then receive loads (as we love our readers so much :) of our great books, content and audio direct to your email account, 100% free!

Get Loads of FREE Stuff at:

https://free.xspurts.com

Chapter One

Introduction to Shiatsu

Shiatsu is a form of massage therapy that originated in Japan and is rooted in the principles of Traditional Chinese Medicine (TCM). This therapy involves applying pressure to specific points on the body to stimulate energy flow and promote physical and emotional well-being. The word "shiatsu" itself means "finger pressure," which refers to the techniques used in this therapy.

Shiatsu is based on the belief that the human body contains a vital energy force known as "qi" or "ki" in Japanese. According to TCM, this energy flows through meridians or channels that run throughout the body. Shiatsu aims to balance and enhance the flow of energy through these channels by applying pressure to specific points, or "tsubos," on the body.

One of the key principles of Shiatsu is that the body and mind are interconnected. Therefore, this therapy not only addresses physical symptoms but also considers emotional and psychological factors. By stimulating the flow of energy through the body, Shiatsu aims to promote relaxation, reduce stress, and improve overall health and well-being.

Shiatsu is often performed on a mat or futon on the floor, and the recipient remains fully clothed. The therapist uses their fingers, thumbs, palms, and elbows to apply pressure to the tsubos, as well as to stretch and manipulate the body. The pressure applied can range from gentle to firm, depending on the individual's needs and preferences.

Shiatsu is known for its ability to alleviate a wide range of physical and emotional conditions. It is particularly effective for relieving muscular tension, reducing pain, and improving circulation. It can also help to boost the immune system, improve digestion, and promote better sleep.

In addition to its physical benefits, Shiatsu is also known for its ability to promote emotional well-being. Many people report feeling a sense of deep relaxation and calmness after a Shiatsu session. This therapy can help to reduce stress and anxiety, improve mood, and promote a sense of overall balance and harmony.

Shiatsu is a highly adaptable therapy that can be tailored to meet the needs of each individual. It can be used as a standalone treatment or as a complement to other forms of healthcare. Many people find Shiatsu to be a valuable part of their self-care routine, as it provides a safe and natural way to promote health and well-being.

Shiatsu has gained popularity around the world, and today, it is practiced by thousands of trained therapists. In Japan, Shiatsu is recognized as a legitimate form of medical treatment and is often covered by health insurance. In other parts of the world, including the United States and Europe, Shiatsu is widely available as an alternative or complementary therapy.

Origins and history

Shiatsu, a form of massage therapy that originated in Japan, has a rich and fascinating history. This therapy has evolved over thousands of years, drawing upon the principles of Traditional Chinese Medicine (TCM) and incorporating elements of Japanese culture and philosophy.

The roots of Shiatsu can be traced back to ancient China, where Traditional Chinese Medicine was first developed. TCM is based on the idea that the human body contains a vital energy force known as "qi" or "ki" in Japanese. This energy flows through meridians or channels that run throughout the body. In TCM, illness and disease are thought to be caused by an imbalance or blockage in the flow of qi.

The practice of Shiatsu emerged in Japan in the early 20th century, although its origins can be traced back to the ancient Japanese art of anma, or massage. Anma was a popular form of therapy in Japan, and it was used to treat a wide range of physical and emotional conditions.

In the early 20th century, a man named Tokujiro Namikoshi began developing a new form of massage therapy that he called "shiatsu." Namikoshi was born in 1905 in Hokkaido, Japan, and he was the son of an anma practitioner. As a child, he suffered from a number of health problems, including pneumonia and tuberculosis. His mother treated him with anma, which inspired his interest in massage therapy.

Namikoshi began developing his own approach to massage therapy in the 1920s. He was particularly interested in the idea of using pressure to stimulate energy flow in the body. Namikoshi believed that this approach could be used to treat a wide range of physical and emotional conditions, and he began teaching his techniques to others.

In 1940, Namikoshi founded the Japan Shiatsu College, which was the first institution dedicated to the study and practice of Shiatsu. The college became a hub for Shiatsu practitioners and helped to popularize the therapy throughout Japan.

Over the decades that followed, Shiatsu continued to evolve and grow in popularity. It was used to treat a wide range of conditions, including musculoskeletal pain, digestive disorders, and emotional imbalances.

In the 1950s, Shiatsu began to gain recognition in the West. Several Westerners traveled to Japan to study the therapy and brought it back to their own countries. In the 1970s, Shiatsu gained further recognition in the United States, where it was embraced as an alternative or complementary therapy.

Today, Shiatsu is practiced all over the world and is recognized as a legitimate form of medical treatment in Japan. It has gained popularity among people seeking natural, non-invasive forms of healthcare and is often used in conjunction with other therapies, such as acupuncture and herbal medicine.

Shiatsu has continued to evolve in recent years, with new techniques and approaches being developed. Some practitioners incorporate elements of Western massage therapy, such as deep tissue massage and myofascial release, into their Shiatsu practice. Others focus more on the traditional techniques and principles of Shiatsu, such as pressure point therapy and energy balancing.

Despite its evolution over the years, Shiatsu remains rooted in the principles of TCM and the ancient wisdom of Japanese culture. It offers a safe, natural, and effective way to promote health and well-being and is a valuable tool for anyone seeking to enhance their quality of life.

Principles and philosophy

Shiatsu is a form of massage therapy that is based on the principles of Traditional Chinese Medicine (TCM) and incorporates elements of Japanese culture and philosophy. At the core of Shiatsu are several key principles that guide its practice and underpin its philosophy.

One of the key principles of Shiatsu is the concept of qi, or vital energy. According to TCM, qi flows through the body along meridians or channels, and its balance and flow are essential for good health. Shiatsu aims to stimulate the flow of qi and promote its balance by applying pressure to specific points on the body.

Another important principle of Shiatsu is the idea of yin and yang, which are opposing yet complementary forces that exist in all things. In TCM, health is thought to depend on a balance between yin and yang. Shiatsu aims to promote this balance by addressing imbalances and blockages in the flow of qi.

Shiatsu also incorporates the concept of the five elements, which are wood, fire, earth, metal, and water. Each element is associated with specific organs, emotions, and other aspects of the body and mind. Shiatsu practitioners use this knowledge to tailor their treatments to the individual needs of each client.

In addition to its principles rooted in TCM, Shiatsu also incorporates elements of Japanese culture and philosophy. One such element is the concept of "hara," which refers to the area around the navel. In Japanese culture, the hara is considered the center of the body and the source of one's energy and vitality. Shiatsu practitioners often focus on the hara during their treatments, using techniques such as abdominal massage to promote relaxation and balance.

Shiatsu also emphasizes the importance of mindfulness and presence during treatments. Practitioners aim to cultivate a state of "ki-ai," which is a focused and attentive state of mind. This helps to promote a deep connection between the practitioner and client and allows the practitioner to work with greater sensitivity and intuition.

Shiatsu vs other massage techniques

Shiatsu is a form of massage therapy that is distinct from other massage techniques in several ways. While all forms of massage involve applying pressure and manipulation to the body, Shiatsu has its own unique set of principles and techniques that set it apart from other modalities.

One of the main differences between Shiatsu and other massage techniques is the way that pressure is applied. In Shiatsu, pressure is applied using the fingers, thumbs, palms, and elbows, and it is focused on specific points or "tsubos" on the body. The pressure applied in Shiatsu can range from gentle to firm, depending on the needs of the individual.

In contrast, many other massage techniques involve a more generalized approach to pressure and manipulation. For example, Swedish massage, which is one of the most popular forms of massage in the West, typically involves long strokes and kneading of the muscles, rather than focusing on specific points.

Another difference between Shiatsu and other massage techniques is the way that the body is positioned during the treatment. In Shiatsu, the recipient typically lies on a mat or futon on the floor, while the practitioner applies pressure using their hands, fingers, and elbows. The recipient remains fully clothed throughout the treatment.

In contrast, many other massage techniques involve the recipient lying on a massage table, often undressed and covered with a sheet or blanket. The practitioner may use oils or lotions to facilitate the massage and may use their whole body to apply pressure, rather than just their hands and fingers.

Shiatsu also differs from other massage techniques in its focus on energy flow and balance. As noted earlier, Shiatsu is based on the principles of Traditional Chinese Medicine, which holds that the body contains a vital energy force known as "qi." Shiatsu aims to stimulate the flow of qi through the body and balance its flow by applying pressure to specific points.

In contrast, many other massage techniques focus primarily on the physical body and its musculature. While some forms of massage, such as Thai massage, may incorporate elements of energy work, they are not based on the same principles as Shiatsu and may have a different focus.

Despite these differences, there are also similarities between Shiatsu and other massage techniques. For example, both Shiatsu and Swedish massage can be used to relieve muscular tension and promote relaxation. Both techniques can also be tailored to the individual needs and preferences of each client.

Similarly, both Shiatsu and Thai massage can be used to stimulate energy flow and promote balance in the body. While the techniques used in these modalities may differ, their underlying principles are similar in many ways.

Chapter Two

Understanding Meridians

Meridians are channels that run throughout the body and are believed to be an integral part of Traditional Chinese Medicine (TCM). These meridians are thought to carry vital energy or "qi" throughout the body, and their balance and flow are essential for good health. In Shiatsu, the meridians are a key element of the therapy, and understanding their function is essential for practitioners and clients alike.

There are 12 primary meridians in the body, each of which is associated with a specific organ system. For example, the lung meridian is associated with the respiratory system, while the liver meridian is associated with the digestive system.

In addition to these primary meridians, there are also eight "extraordinary" meridians, which are not associated with a specific organ system but are believed to play a vital role in overall health and well-being.

The meridians are not visible to the naked eye, and their existence cannot be proven through conventional scientific methods. However, they are widely accepted in TCM and other forms of alternative medicine as a key element of the body's energy system.

Shiatsu practitioners use their knowledge of the meridians to tailor their treatments to the individual needs of each client. By applying pressure to specific points along the meridians, they aim to stimulate the flow of qi and promote its balance throughout the body.

One of the key concepts in understanding meridians is the idea of "acupoints." Acupoints are specific points along the meridians where pressure can be applied to promote the flow of qi. In Shiatsu, these acupoints are known as "tsubos," and they are the focus of the therapy.

The acupoints along the meridians are believed to have specific functions and properties. For example, some acupoints may be used to promote relaxation and reduce stress, while others may be used to alleviate pain or improve digestion.

Shiatsu practitioners use their knowledge of the acupoints to develop a treatment plan that is tailored to the individual needs of each client. By identifying the specific acupoints that are most relevant to the client's condition, they can apply pressure in a targeted and effective way.

While the concept of meridians may seem unfamiliar to those who are accustomed to Western medicine, it is important to recognize that many of the concepts that underpin TCM have been validated by scientific research. For example, studies have shown that acupuncture, which is another form of therapy that is based on the meridian system, can be effective in treating a wide range of conditions, from pain and inflammation to anxiety and depression.

In addition to its potential therapeutic benefits, the concept of meridians can also be helpful in understanding the body's energy system and its interconnections. By recognizing the interconnectedness of the various organ systems and energy pathways in the body, we can gain a deeper understanding of the complex processes that underlie health and well-being.

The concept of Ki (energy)

In Shiatsu, the concept of "ki," or vital energy, is central to the therapy. Ki is a fundamental concept in Traditional Chinese Medicine (TCM) and is believed to flow through the body along meridians or channels. The balance and flow of ki are essential for good health, and Shiatsu aims to promote this balance by stimulating the flow of ki through the body.

The concept of ki is rooted in the ancient philosophy of Taoism, which holds that everything in the universe is made up of energy or "qi." In TCM, this concept is applied to the human body, where ki is thought to flow through the meridians and provide the body with the energy it needs to function properly.

Ki is not visible to the naked eye, and its existence cannot be proven through conventional scientific methods. However, it is widely accepted in TCM and other forms of alternative medicine as a vital component of the body's energy system.

Shiatsu practitioners use their knowledge of ki to tailor their treatments to the individual needs of each client. By stimulating the flow of ki through the body, they aim to promote its balance and restore health and vitality.

One of the key concepts in understanding ki is the idea of yin and yang. Yin and yang are opposing yet complementary forces that exist in all things, including the human body. In TCM, health is thought to depend on a balance between yin and yang, and Shiatsu aims to promote this balance by addressing imbalances and blockages in the flow of ki.

Another important concept in understanding ki is the idea of "hara." In Japanese culture, the hara is considered the center of the body and the source of one's energy and vitality. Shiatsu practitioners often focus on the hara during their treatments, using techniques such as abdominal massage to promote relaxation and balance.

Shiatsu also emphasizes the importance of mindfulness and presence during treatments. Practitioners aim to cultivate a state of "ki-ai," which is a focused and attentive state of mind. This helps to promote a deep connection between the practitioner and client and allows the practitioner to work with greater sensitivity and intuition.

While the concept of ki may be unfamiliar to those who are accustomed to Western medicine, it is important to recognize that many of the concepts that underpin TCM have been validated by scientific research. For example, studies have shown that acupuncture, which is another form of therapy that is based on the concept of ki, can be effective in treating a wide range of conditions, from pain and inflammation to anxiety and depression.

In addition to its potential therapeutic benefits, the concept of ki can also be helpful in understanding the body's energy system and its interconnections. By recognizing the interconnectedness of the various organ systems and energy pathways in the body, we can gain a deeper understanding of the complex processes that underlie health and well-being.

The 12 main meridians

Shiatsu is a form of massage therapy that is based on the principles of Traditional Chinese Medicine (TCM) and incorporates elements of Japanese culture and philosophy. At the core of Shiatsu are the meridians, or channels, that run throughout the body and are believed to carry vital energy or "qi." Understanding the 12 main meridians is essential for Shiatsu practitioners, as they use their knowledge of these channels to tailor their treatments to the individual needs of each client.

1. Lung Meridian: The lung meridian runs from the chest down to the hand and is associated with the respiratory system. Shiatsu techniques

that stimulate the lung meridian can be helpful in relieving breathing difficulties, coughing, and other respiratory problems.

2. Large Intestine Meridian: The large intestine meridian runs from the hand up to the face and is associated with the digestive system. Shiatsu techniques that stimulate the large intestine meridian can be helpful in relieving constipation, diarrhea, and other digestive problems.

3. Stomach Meridian: The stomach meridian runs from the face down to the foot and is associated with the digestive system. Shiatsu techniques that stimulate the stomach meridian can be helpful in relieving nausea, vomiting, and other digestive problems.

4. Spleen Meridian: The spleen meridian runs from the foot up to the chest and is associated with the digestive system. Shiatsu techniques that stimulate the spleen meridian can be helpful in relieving bloating, gas, and other digestive problems.

5. Heart Meridian: The heart meridian runs from the chest down to the hand and is associated with the circulatory system. Shiatsu techniques that stimulate the heart meridian can be helpful in relieving chest pain, high blood pressure, and other circulatory problems.

6. Small Intestine Meridian: The small intestine meridian runs from the hand up to the ear and is associated with the digestive system. Shiatsu techniques that stimulate the small intestine meridian can be helpful in relieving bloating, gas, and other digestive problems.

7. Bladder Meridian: The bladder meridian runs from the foot up to the head and is associated with the urinary system. Shiatsu techniques that stimulate the bladder meridian can be helpful in relieving urinary incontinence, bladder infections, and other urinary problems.

8. Kidney Meridian: The kidney meridian runs from the foot up to the chest and is associated with the urinary system. Shiatsu techniques that stimulate the kidney meridian can be helpful in relieving urinary incontinence, kidney infections, and other urinary problems.

9. Pericardium Meridian: The pericardium meridian runs from the chest down to the hand and is associated with the circulatory system. Shiatsu techniques that stimulate the pericardium meridian can be helpful in relieving chest pain, palpitations, and other circulatory problems.

10. Triple Warmer Meridian: The triple warmer meridian runs from the hand up to the face and is associated with the nervous system. Shiatsu techniques that stimulate the triple warmer meridian can be helpful in relieving anxiety, stress, and other nervous system problems.

11. Gallbladder Meridian: The gallbladder meridian runs from the face down to the foot and is associated with the digestive system. Shiatsu techniques that stimulate the gallbladder meridian can be helpful in relieving digestive problems and liver disorders.

12. Liver Meridian: The liver meridian runs from the foot up to the chest and is associated with the digestive system. Shiatsu techniques that stimulate the liver meridian can be helpful in relieving liver disorders, digestive problems, and emotional issues.

Meridian functions and associations

Meridians are channels that run throughout the body and are believed to be an integral part of Traditional Chinese Medicine (TCM). These meridians are thought to carry vital energy or "qi" throughout the body, and their balance and flow are essential for good health. In Shiatsu, the meridians are a key element of the therapy, and understanding their functions and associations is essential for practitioners and clients alike.

Each of the 12 main meridians in the body is associated with a specific organ system or function. By understanding the functions and associations of these meridians, Shiatsu practitioners can develop treatments that are tailored to the individual needs of each client.

1. Lung Meridian: The lung meridian is associated with the respiratory system and is responsible for regulating breathing and the immune system. Shiatsu techniques that stimulate the lung meridian can be helpful in relieving breathing difficulties and boosting the immune system.

2. Large Intestine Meridian: The large intestine meridian is associated with the digestive system and is responsible for the absorption and elimination of food. Shiatsu techniques that stimulate the large intestine meridian can be helpful in relieving constipation, diarrhea, and other digestive problems.

3. Stomach Meridian: The stomach meridian is associated with the digestive system and is responsible for breaking down and digesting food. Shiatsu techniques that stimulate the stomach meridian can be helpful in relieving nausea, vomiting, and other digestive problems.

4. Spleen Meridian: The spleen meridian is associated with the digestive system and is responsible for filtering blood and regulating blood sugar levels. Shiatsu techniques that stimulate the spleen meridian can be helpful in relieving bloating, gas, and other digestive problems.

5. Heart Meridian: The heart meridian is associated with the circulatory system and is responsible for regulating blood flow and circulation. Shiatsu techniques that stimulate the heart meridian can be helpful in relieving chest pain, high blood pressure, and other circulatory problems.

6. Small Intestine Meridian: The small intestine meridian is associated with the digestive system and is responsible for breaking down food and absorbing nutrients. Shiatsu techniques that stimulate the small intestine meridian can be helpful in relieving bloating, gas, and other digestive problems.

7. Bladder Meridian: The bladder meridian is associated with the urinary system and is responsible for regulating urine flow and eliminating waste products from the body. Shiatsu techniques that stimulate the bladder meridian can be helpful in relieving urinary incontinence, bladder infections, and other urinary problems.

8. Kidney Meridian: The kidney meridian is associated with the urinary system and is responsible for regulating urine production and maintaining fluid balance in the body. Shiatsu techniques that stimulate the kidney meridian can be helpful in relieving urinary incontinence, kidney infections, and other urinary problems.

9. Pericardium Meridian: The pericardium meridian is associated with the circulatory system and is responsible for regulating blood flow and circulation. Shiatsu techniques that stimulate the pericardium meridian can be helpful in relieving chest pain, palpitations, and other circulatory problems.

10. Triple Warmer Meridian: The triple warmer meridian is associated with the nervous system and is responsible for regulating the body's response to stress and other stimuli. Shiatsu techniques that stimulate the triple warmer meridian can be helpful in relieving anxiety, stress, and other nervous system problems.

11. Gallbladder Meridian: The gallbladder meridian is associated with the digestive system and is responsible for the storage and secretion of bile.

Shiatsu techniques that stimulate the gallbladder meridian can be helpful in relieving digestive problems and liver disorders.

Liver Meridian

Chapter Three

Basic Techniques of Shiatsu

Shiatsu is a form of massage therapy that is based on the principles of Traditional Chinese Medicine (TCM) and incorporates elements of Japanese culture and philosophy. The aim of Shiatsu is to promote the balance and flow of vital energy or "qi" throughout the body, which is believed to be essential for good health. Shiatsu practitioners use a range of techniques to stimulate the body's energy system and promote relaxation and healing.

1. Pressure Points: One of the most fundamental techniques in Shiatsu is the use of pressure points. Pressure points are specific areas of the body where the flow of energy is believed to be concentrated. By applying pressure to these points, Shiatsu practitioners can stimulate the flow of energy and promote relaxation and healing.

2. Palming: Palming is a technique where the practitioner uses their palms to apply pressure to the body. This technique can be used to stimulate the flow of energy and promote relaxation and healing.

3. Kneading: Kneading is a technique where the practitioner uses their fingers and thumbs to knead and manipulate the muscles and soft tissue of the body. This technique can be used to relieve tension and promote relaxation.

4. Stretching: Stretching is a technique where the practitioner gently stretches and manipulates the muscles and soft tissue of the body. This technique can be used to increase flexibility and promote relaxation.

5. Rocking: Rocking is a technique where the practitioner gently rocks the body back and forth. This technique can be used to promote relaxation and a sense of calm.

6. Rotation: Rotation is a technique where the practitioner rotates and manipulates the joints of the body. This technique can be used to relieve tension and promote relaxation.

7. Tapping: Tapping is a technique where the practitioner uses their fingers and hands to tap and massage the body. This technique can be used to stimulate the flow of energy and promote relaxation.

8. Vibration: Vibration is a technique where the practitioner uses their hands or a special tool to create a vibrating sensation on the body. This technique can be used to stimulate the flow of energy and promote relaxation.

9. Finger Pressure: Finger pressure is a technique where the practitioner uses their fingers to apply pressure to specific areas of the body. This technique can be used to stimulate the flow of energy and promote relaxation.

10. Acupressure: Acupressure is a technique where the practitioner uses their fingers to apply pressure to specific acupuncture points on the body. This technique can be used to stimulate the flow of energy and promote relaxation.

Finger pressure

Finger pressure is a fundamental technique used in Shiatsu massage therapy. Shiatsu is a form of massage therapy based on the principles of Traditional Chinese Medicine (TCM) and Japanese culture and philosophy. The technique involves applying pressure with the fingers to specific points on the body, which are believed to correspond to various organs and systems. This technique is based on the principles of acupressure, which is an ancient healing method that has been used for thousands of years.

Finger pressure is a powerful technique that can be used to promote healing, reduce stress, and alleviate pain. It is a non-invasive method that can be used to treat a variety of conditions, including headaches, back pain, digestive problems, and anxiety. Finger pressure works by stimulating the flow of energy or "qi" throughout the body, which is believed to be essential for good health.

Shiatsu practitioners use their fingers to apply pressure to specific points on the body, known as acupressure points. These points are located along the meridians, or energy channels, that run throughout the body. Each point corresponds to a specific organ or system in the body, and by applying pressure to these points, the flow of energy can be stimulated, promoting relaxation and healing.

One of the primary benefits of finger pressure is its ability to relieve tension and promote relaxation. By applying pressure to specific points on the body, Shiatsu practitioners can help to release tension and promote a sense of calm and relaxation. This technique can be particularly helpful for individuals who are experiencing stress, anxiety, or other emotional issues.

Another benefit of finger pressure is its ability to alleviate pain. By stimulating the flow of energy throughout the body, Shiatsu practitioners can help to relieve pain and discomfort caused by a variety of conditions, including headaches, back pain, and menstrual cramps.

Finger pressure can also be used to improve the functioning of various organs and systems in the body. By applying pressure to specific points, Shiatsu practitioners can help to promote the flow of energy to these areas, which can help to improve the functioning of the corresponding organs and systems.

It is important to note that finger pressure should always be performed by a trained and licensed Shiatsu practitioner. While finger pressure is generally considered to be safe, it is important to receive treatment from a qualified practitioner who has undergone extensive training in the technique.

Palm pressure

Palm pressure is a technique used in Shiatsu massage therapy that involves using the palms of the hands to apply pressure to specific points on the body. Shiatsu is a form of massage therapy that is based on the principles of Traditional Chinese Medicine (TCM) and Japanese culture and philosophy. The technique aims to promote the balance and flow of vital energy or "qi" throughout the body, which is believed to be essential for good health.

Palm pressure is a gentle yet powerful technique that can be used to promote relaxation, reduce stress, and alleviate pain. It is a non-invasive method that can be used to treat a variety of conditions, including headaches, back pain, and digestive problems. The technique involves using the palms of the hands to apply pressure to specific points on the body, which are believed to correspond to various organs and systems.

One of the primary benefits of palm pressure is its ability to promote relaxation. By applying pressure with the palms of the hands, Shiatsu practitioners can help to release tension and promote a sense of calm and relaxation. This technique can be particularly helpful for individuals who are experiencing stress or anxiety.

Another benefit of palm pressure is its ability to alleviate pain. By stimulating the flow of energy throughout the body, Shiatsu practitioners can help to relieve pain and discomfort caused by a variety of conditions, including headaches, back pain, and menstrual cramps.

Palm pressure can also be used to improve the functioning of various organs and systems in the body. By applying pressure to specific points, Shiatsu practitioners can help to promote the flow of energy to these areas, which can help to improve the functioning of the corresponding organs and systems.

It is important to note that palm pressure should always be performed by a trained and licensed Shiatsu practitioner. While palm pressure is generally considered to be safe, it is important to receive treatment from a qualified practitioner who has undergone extensive training in the technique.

In addition to promoting relaxation and pain relief, palm pressure can also have a positive impact on mental and emotional well-being. By stimulating the flow of energy throughout the body, Shiatsu practitioners can help to promote a sense of balance and harmony, which can improve mood and reduce feelings of anxiety and depression.

Kneading

Kneading is a technique used in Shiatsu massage therapy that involves manipulating the muscles and soft tissue of the body with the fingers and thumbs. Shiatsu is a form of massage therapy that is based on the principles of Traditional Chinese Medicine (TCM) and Japanese culture and philosophy. The technique aims to promote the balance and flow of vital energy or "qi" throughout the body, which is believed to be essential for good health.

Kneading is a powerful technique that can be used to relieve tension and promote relaxation. It involves using the fingers and thumbs to apply pressure to the muscles and soft tissue of the body, which can help to relieve tightness and promote a sense of calm and relaxation. Kneading can be particularly effective for individuals who are experiencing stress or anxiety.

One of the primary benefits of kneading is its ability to relieve pain. By manipulating the muscles and soft tissue of the body, Shiatsu practitioners can help to relieve pain and discomfort caused by a variety of conditions, including headaches, back pain, and menstrual cramps. The technique can be used to improve circulation, increase flexibility, and reduce inflammation, which can help to alleviate pain and promote healing.

Kneading can also be used to improve the functioning of various organs and systems in the body. By manipulating the muscles and soft tissue of the body, Shiatsu practitioners can help to promote the flow of energy to these areas, which can help to improve the functioning of the corresponding organs and systems.

It is important to note that kneading should always be performed by a trained and licensed Shiatsu practitioner. While kneading is generally considered to be safe, it is important to receive treatment from a qualified practitioner who has undergone extensive training in the technique.

In addition to promoting relaxation and pain relief, kneading can also have a positive impact on mental and emotional well-being. By promoting the flow of energy throughout the body, Shiatsu practitioners can help to promote a sense of balance and harmony, which can improve mood and reduce feelings of anxiety and depression.

Stretching

Stretching is a technique used in Shiatsu massage therapy that involves gently manipulating the muscles and soft tissue of the body to increase flexibility and promote relaxation. Shiatsu is a form of massage therapy that is based on the principles of Traditional Chinese Medicine (TCM) and Japanese culture and philosophy. The technique aims to promote the balance and flow of vital energy or "qi" throughout the body, which is believed to be essential for good health.

Stretching is a powerful technique that can be used to improve flexibility and reduce tension. It involves gently manipulating the muscles and soft tissue of the body to promote relaxation and increase mobility. Stretching can be particularly effective for individuals who are experiencing stiffness or limited mobility.

One of the primary benefits of stretching is its ability to promote relaxation. By gently manipulating the muscles and soft tissue of the body, Shiatsu practitioners can help to release tension and promote a sense of calm and relaxation. This technique can be particularly helpful for individuals who are experiencing stress or anxiety.

Another benefit of stretching is its ability to improve flexibility. By gently stretching and manipulating the muscles and soft tissue of the body, Shiatsu practitioners can help to increase mobility and improve flexibility. This can be particularly beneficial for individuals who are experiencing stiffness or limited mobility.

Stretching can also be used to improve the functioning of various organs and systems in the body. By gently manipulating the muscles and soft tissue of the body, Shiatsu practitioners can help to promote the flow of energy to these areas, which can help to improve the functioning of the corresponding organs and systems.

It is important to note that stretching should always be performed by a trained and licensed Shiatsu practitioner. While stretching is generally considered to be safe, it is important to receive treatment from a qualified practitioner who has undergone extensive training in the technique.

In addition to promoting relaxation and increasing flexibility, stretching can also have a positive impact on mental and emotional well-being. By promoting the flow of energy throughout the body, Shiatsu practitioners can help to promote a sense of balance and harmony, which can improve mood and reduce feelings of anxiety and depression.

Chapter Four

Practicing Proper Body Mechanics

Practicing proper body mechanics is essential for anyone working in the field of Shiatsu massage therapy. Shiatsu is a form of massage therapy that is based on the principles of Traditional Chinese Medicine (TCM) and Japanese culture and philosophy. The technique involves applying pressure to specific points on the body, which can help to promote relaxation, relieve pain, and improve overall health and wellness.

Proper body mechanics involve the correct use of the body to perform tasks safely and efficiently. In the context of Shiatsu massage therapy, this means using proper posture, positioning, and movement to ensure that both the practitioner and the client are safe and comfortable during treatment.

One of the most important aspects of proper body mechanics is maintaining good posture. This means standing up straight, with the shoulders back and the chest open. Good posture helps to prevent strain on the back and neck, which can be a common problem for massage therapists who spend long hours working in a bent-over position.

Another important aspect of proper body mechanics is using the legs and arms to lift and move the client's body. This helps to distribute the weight evenly across the body, reducing the risk of injury or strain. It is also important to avoid twisting or bending the body while lifting or moving the client.

Shiatsu practitioners should also be aware of their breathing and movement patterns. It is important to breathe deeply and naturally, using the diaphragm to expand the lungs and promote relaxation. Practitioners should also avoid jerky or sudden movements, instead using slow, smooth movements to apply pressure to specific points on the body.

In addition to using proper posture and movement techniques, Shiatsu practitioners should also be aware of their surroundings. This includes making sure that the treatment room is clean, well-lit, and free from clutter or obstacles. Practitioners should also be aware of any potential hazards, such as uneven flooring or sharp objects, and take steps to minimize the risk of injury.

Finally, it is important for Shiatsu practitioners to take care of their own health and well-being. This means getting enough rest, staying hydrated, and engaging in regular exercise and stretching. Practitioners should also be aware of their own physical limitations and avoid pushing themselves too hard during treatment.

Posture and alignment

Posture and alignment are important considerations in Shiatsu massage therapy. Shiatsu is a form of massage therapy that is based on the principles of Traditional Chinese Medicine (TCM) and Japanese culture and philosophy. The technique involves applying pressure to specific points on the body, which can help to promote relaxation, relieve pain, and improve overall health and wellness.

Proper posture and alignment are important for both the practitioner and the client during Shiatsu massage therapy. Good posture helps to prevent strain on the back and neck, which can be a common problem for massage therapists who spend long hours working in a bent-over position. Proper alignment helps to ensure that the body is in balance, with the muscles, bones, and joints working together effectively.

One of the most important aspects of proper posture and alignment is maintaining good spinal alignment. This means keeping the spine in a neutral position, with the natural curves of the spine supported by the muscles and ligaments. The shoulders should be relaxed and the chest should be open, allowing for proper breathing and circulation.

Another important aspect of proper posture and alignment is maintaining a stable base of support. This means keeping the feet hip-width apart and planting them firmly on the ground. The knees should be slightly bent and the weight should be evenly distributed between the feet.

Shiatsu practitioners should also be aware of their own body mechanics during treatment. This means using proper posture and movement techniques to avoid strain on the back, neck, and other areas of the body. Practitioners should also be aware of their breathing and movement patterns, using slow, smooth movements to apply pressure to specific points on the body.

In addition to proper posture and alignment during treatment, Shiatsu practitioners should also encourage their clients to maintain good posture and alignment throughout their daily lives. This includes sitting and standing with the spine in a neutral position, using proper ergonomics at work and at home, and engaging in regular exercise and stretching.

Improper posture and alignment can lead to a variety of health problems, including back pain, neck pain, and headaches. By maintaining good posture and alignment, Shiatsu practitioners can help to prevent these problems and promote overall health and well-being.

Breathing techniques

Breathing techniques are an important component of Shiatsu massage therapy. Shiatsu is a form of massage therapy that is based on the principles of Traditional Chinese Medicine (TCM) and Japanese culture and philosophy. The technique involves applying pressure to specific points on the body, which can help to promote relaxation, relieve pain, and improve overall health and wellness.

Proper breathing techniques are essential for both the practitioner and the client during Shiatsu massage therapy. Breathing deeply and naturally helps to promote relaxation, reduce stress, and increase the flow of vital energy or "qi" throughout the body.

One of the primary goals of Shiatsu massage therapy is to promote the flow of qi throughout the body. Breathing deeply and naturally can help to facilitate this process, allowing the body to relax and the energy to flow freely.

During Shiatsu massage therapy, both the practitioner and the client should focus on breathing deeply and naturally. This means inhaling deeply through the nose, filling the lungs with air, and exhaling slowly through the mouth. The breath should be slow, smooth, and rhythmic, allowing the body to relax and the mind to become calm.

Shiatsu practitioners should also be aware of their own breathing patterns during treatment. It is important to breathe deeply and naturally, using the diaphragm to expand the lungs and promote relaxation. Practitioners should also avoid holding their breath or breathing shallowly, which can cause tension and discomfort in the body.

In addition to promoting relaxation and the flow of qi, proper breathing techniques can also have a positive impact on mental and emotional well-being. By focusing on the breath and maintaining a slow, smooth, and rhythmic pattern, individuals can reduce feelings of anxiety, stress, and depression, and promote a sense of calm and well-being.

Using your body weight effectively

Using your body weight effectively is an important consideration in Shiatsu massage therapy. Shiatsu is a form of massage therapy that is based on the principles of Traditional Chinese Medicine (TCM) and Japanese culture and philosophy. The technique involves applying pressure to specific points on the body, which can help to promote relaxation, relieve pain, and improve overall health and wellness.

Using your body weight effectively means using the weight of your body to apply pressure to the client's body, rather than relying solely on the strength of your hands and arms. This allows the practitioner to apply deep pressure without causing strain or discomfort in their hands or wrists.

One of the primary benefits of using your body weight effectively is that it allows you to apply deep pressure to specific points on the body. Deep pressure can be particularly effective for individuals who are experiencing chronic pain or tension, and can help to promote relaxation and reduce discomfort.

To use your body weight effectively during Shiatsu massage therapy, it is important to maintain good posture and alignment. This means standing up straight, with the shoulders back and the chest open. The feet should be hip-width apart and planted firmly on the ground, with the knees slightly bent.

It is also important to use your legs and core muscles to generate force, rather than relying solely on the strength of your arms and hands. This means engaging the muscles in your legs and core, and using your body weight to apply pressure to the client's body.

Shiatsu practitioners should also be aware of their own body mechanics during treatment. This means using proper posture and movement techniques to avoid strain on the back, neck, and other areas of the body. Practitioners should also be aware of their breathing and movement patterns, using slow, smooth movements to apply pressure to specific points on the body.

In addition to using your body weight effectively, it is also important to communicate with the client during treatment. This includes asking for feedback about the pressure and intensity of the massage, and making adjustments as necessary. It is also important to check in with the client regularly to ensure that they are comfortable and relaxed throughout the treatment.

Chapter Five

Shiatsu for Common Ailments

Shiatsu massage therapy can be an effective treatment option for a wide range of common ailments. Shiatsu is a form of massage therapy that is based on the principles of Traditional Chinese Medicine (TCM) and Japanese culture and philosophy. The technique involves applying pressure to specific points on the body, which can help to promote relaxation, relieve pain, and improve overall health and wellness.

Here are some common ailments that Shiatsu massage therapy can be used to treat:

1. Back pain: Shiatsu massage therapy can be an effective treatment option for individuals who are experiencing back pain. By applying pressure to specific points on the back, Shiatsu massage can help to relieve tension, reduce inflammation, and promote relaxation.

2. Headaches: Shiatsu massage therapy can also be an effective treatment option for individuals who are experiencing headaches. By applying pressure to specific points on the head and neck, Shiatsu massage can help to relieve tension and reduce the frequency and severity of headaches.

3. Insomnia: Shiatsu massage therapy can be an effective treatment option for individuals who are experiencing insomnia or other sleep disturbances. By promoting relaxation and reducing stress, Shiatsu massage can help to improve sleep quality and duration.

4. Stress and anxiety: Shiatsu massage therapy can also be an effective treatment option for individuals who are experiencing stress or anxiety. By promoting relaxation and reducing tension, Shiatsu massage can help to reduce feelings of stress and anxiety, and promote a sense of calm and well-being.

5. Digestive issues: Shiatsu massage therapy can be an effective treatment option for individuals who are experiencing digestive issues, such as bloating, constipation, or diarrhea. By applying pressure to specific points on the abdomen, Shiatsu massage can help to promote healthy digestion and reduce discomfort.

6. Menstrual cramps: Shiatsu massage therapy can also be an effective treatment option for individuals who are experiencing menstrual cramps. By applying pressure to specific points on the abdomen and lower back, Shiatsu massage can help to reduce pain and discomfort associated with menstrual cramps.

7. Respiratory issues: Shiatsu massage therapy can be an effective treatment option for individuals who are experiencing respiratory issues, such as asthma or allergies. By promoting relaxation and reducing tension in the muscles surrounding the lungs, Shiatsu massage can help to improve breathing and reduce symptoms.

Headaches and migraines

Headaches and migraines are a common ailment that affects millions of people worldwide. Shiatsu massage therapy can be an effective treatment option for individuals who are experiencing headaches or migraines. Shiatsu is a form of massage therapy that is based on the principles of Traditional Chinese Medicine (TCM) and Japanese culture and philosophy. The technique involves applying pressure to specific points on the body, which can help to promote relaxation, relieve pain, and improve overall health and wellness.

Headaches and migraines are often caused by tension and stress in the muscles of the head, neck, and shoulders. Shiatsu massage therapy can be effective in relieving tension in these muscles, reducing the frequency and severity of headaches and migraines.

During Shiatsu massage therapy for headaches and migraines, the practitioner will focus on applying pressure to specific points on the head, neck, and shoulders. These points are often located in areas where tension is commonly held, such as the temples, base of the skull, and along the spine.

Shiatsu massage therapy for headaches and migraines may also involve stretching and gentle manipulation of the neck and shoulders. This can help to release tension and improve range of motion, which can also help to reduce the frequency and severity of headaches and migraines.

In addition to Shiatsu massage therapy, there are also lifestyle changes that individuals can make to reduce the frequency and severity of headaches and migraines. These include:

1. Managing stress: Stress is a common trigger for headaches and migraines. Engaging in stress-reducing activities such as meditation, yoga, or deep breathing exercises can help to reduce stress and prevent headaches and migraines.

2. Getting enough sleep: Lack of sleep can also be a trigger for headaches and migraines. It is important to get enough sleep each night to help prevent these types of headaches.

3. Staying hydrated: Dehydration can also be a trigger for headaches and migraines. It is important to drink plenty of water throughout the day to stay hydrated.

4. Eating a healthy diet: Eating a healthy diet can also help to prevent headaches and migraines. Avoiding trigger foods such as caffeine, alcohol, and processed foods can help to reduce the frequency and severity of headaches and migraines.

Back pain

Back pain is a common ailment that affects millions of people worldwide. Shiatsu massage therapy can be an effective treatment option for individuals who are experiencing back pain. Shiatsu is a form of massage therapy that is based on the principles of Traditional Chinese Medicine (TCM) and Japanese culture and philosophy. The technique involves applying pressure to specific points on the body, which can help to promote relaxation, relieve pain, and improve overall health and wellness.

Back pain can be caused by a variety of factors, including poor posture, injury, or tension in the muscles of the back. Shiatsu massage therapy can be effective in relieving tension in these muscles, reducing pain and discomfort associated with back pain.

During Shiatsu massage therapy for back pain, the practitioner will focus on applying pressure to specific points along the spine, as well as other points on the back, hips, and legs. These points are often located in areas where tension is commonly held, such as the lower back, shoulders, and hips.

Shiatsu massage therapy for back pain may also involve stretching and gentle manipulation of the back and hips. This can help to release tension and improve range of motion, which can also help to reduce pain and discomfort associated with back pain.

In addition to Shiatsu massage therapy, there are also lifestyle changes that individuals can make to reduce the frequency and severity of back pain. These include:

1. Maintaining good posture: Poor posture is a common cause of back pain. It is important to maintain good posture throughout the day, especially when sitting or standing for long periods of time.

2. Engaging in regular exercise: Regular exercise can help to strengthen the muscles of the back and improve overall health and wellness. Low-impact exercises such as yoga or swimming can be particularly effective for individuals who are experiencing back pain.

3. Staying hydrated: Dehydration can also contribute to back pain. It is important to drink plenty of water throughout the day to stay hydrated and reduce the risk of back pain.

4. Getting enough sleep: Lack of sleep can also contribute to back pain. It is important to get enough sleep each night to help prevent back pain.

Insomnia

Insomnia is a common sleep disorder that affects millions of people worldwide. Shiatsu massage therapy can be an effective treatment option for individuals who are experiencing insomnia. Shiatsu is a form of massage therapy that is based on the principles of Traditional Chinese Medicine (TCM) and Japanese culture and philosophy. The technique involves applying pressure to specific points on the body, which can help to promote relaxation, relieve pain, and improve overall health and wellness.

Insomnia is often caused by stress, anxiety, or tension in the muscles of the body. Shiatsu massage therapy can be effective in relieving tension in these muscles, promoting relaxation, and improving sleep quality and duration.

During Shiatsu massage therapy for insomnia, the practitioner will focus on applying pressure to specific points on the body that are associated with relaxation and sleep. These points may be located on the head, neck, shoulders, back, and feet.

Shiatsu massage therapy for insomnia may also involve stretching and gentle manipulation of the muscles of the body. This can help to release tension and improve circulation, which can also help to promote relaxation and improve sleep quality.

In addition to Shiatsu massage therapy, there are also lifestyle changes that individuals can make to improve sleep quality and reduce the frequency and severity of insomnia. These include:

1. Establishing a regular sleep routine: It is important to establish a regular sleep routine by going to bed and waking up at the same time each day.

2. Avoiding caffeine and alcohol: Caffeine and alcohol can interfere with sleep quality and contribute to insomnia. It is important to avoid these substances, especially in the hours leading up to bedtime.

3. Engaging in relaxation techniques: Relaxation techniques such as meditation, yoga, or deep breathing exercises can help to reduce stress and promote relaxation, which can improve sleep quality.

4. Creating a comfortable sleep environment: Creating a comfortable sleep environment by ensuring the room is dark, quiet, and at a comfortable temperature can also help to improve sleep quality.

Digestive issues

Digestive issues are a common ailment that affects millions of people worldwide. Shiatsu massage therapy can be an effective treatment option for individuals who are experiencing digestive issues. Shiatsu is a form of massage therapy that is based on the principles of Traditional Chinese Medicine (TCM) and Japanese culture and philosophy. The technique involves applying pressure to specific points on the body, which can help to promote relaxation, relieve pain, and improve overall health and wellness.

Digestive issues can be caused by a variety of factors, including poor diet, stress, and tension in the muscles of the abdomen. Shiatsu massage therapy can be effective in relieving tension in these muscles, promoting relaxation, and improving digestion.

During Shiatsu massage therapy for digestive issues, the practitioner will focus on applying pressure to specific points on the abdomen and along the meridians that are associated with digestion. These points are often located in areas where tension is commonly held, such as the lower abdomen and the area around the navel.

Shiatsu massage therapy for digestive issues may also involve stretching and gentle manipulation of the muscles of the abdomen. This can help to improve circulation and promote relaxation, which can improve digestion.

In addition to Shiatsu massage therapy, there are also lifestyle changes that individuals can make to improve digestion and reduce the frequency and severity of digestive issues. These include:

1. Eating a healthy diet: A healthy diet that is rich in fiber, fruits, and vegetables can help to improve digestion and reduce the risk of digestive issues.

2. Managing stress: Stress can contribute to digestive issues. Engaging in stress-reducing activities such as meditation, yoga, or deep breathing exercises can help to reduce stress and improve digestion.

3. Staying hydrated: Dehydration can also contribute to digestive issues. It is important to drink plenty of water throughout the day to stay hydrated and improve digestion.

4. Engaging in regular exercise: Regular exercise can help to improve digestion and reduce the risk of digestive issues. Low-impact exercises such as yoga or walking can be particularly effective for individuals who are experiencing digestive issues.

Chapter Six

Shiatsu for Stress Relief and Relaxation

Stress is a common issue that affects millions of people worldwide. Shiatsu massage therapy can be an effective treatment option for individuals who are experiencing stress and are looking to promote relaxation. Shiatsu is a form of massage therapy that is based on the principles of Traditional Chinese Medicine (TCM) and Japanese culture and philosophy. The technique involves applying pressure to specific points on the body, which can help to promote relaxation, relieve pain, and improve overall health and wellness.

During Shiatsu massage therapy for stress relief and relaxation, the practitioner will focus on applying pressure to specific points on the body that are associated with relaxation and stress relief. These points may be located on the head, neck, shoulders, back, and feet.

Shiatsu massage therapy for stress relief and relaxation may also involve stretching and gentle manipulation of the muscles of the body. This can help to release tension, improve circulation, and promote relaxation.

Shiatsu massage therapy for stress relief and relaxation can also have a positive impact on the body's nervous system. By promoting relaxation and reducing stress, Shiatsu massage therapy can help to activate the parasympathetic nervous system, which is responsible for promoting relaxation and rest. This can help to improve sleep quality, reduce muscle tension, and improve overall health and wellness.

In addition to Shiatsu massage therapy, there are also lifestyle changes that individuals can make to reduce stress and promote relaxation. These include:

1. Engaging in stress-reducing activities: Engaging in activities that promote relaxation and reduce stress, such as meditation, yoga, or deep breathing exercises, can help to reduce stress and promote relaxation.

2. Getting enough sleep: Lack of sleep can contribute to stress and tension in the body. It is important to get enough sleep each night to promote relaxation and reduce stress.

3. Maintaining a healthy diet: A healthy diet that is rich in fruits, vegetables, and whole grains can help to reduce stress and promote relaxation.

4. Engaging in regular exercise: Regular exercise can help to reduce stress and tension in the body, improve circulation, and promote relaxation.

Techniques to calm the nervous system

The nervous system plays a critical role in regulating various bodily functions, including the stress response, sleep, and digestion. When the nervous system becomes overactive, it can lead to symptoms such as anxiety, restlessness, and insomnia. Shiatsu massage therapy can be an effective treatment option for individuals who are experiencing an overactive nervous system and are looking to promote relaxation. In addition to Shiatsu massage therapy, there are also several techniques that individuals can use to calm the nervous system.

1. Deep breathing exercises: Deep breathing exercises can be an effective technique for calming the nervous system. Deep breathing can help to slow down the heart rate, lower blood pressure, and promote relaxation. To

perform deep breathing exercises, simply inhale deeply through the nose and exhale slowly through the mouth.

2. Progressive muscle relaxation: Progressive muscle relaxation is a technique that involves tensing and relaxing different muscle groups in the body. This technique can help to promote relaxation and reduce tension in the muscles. To perform progressive muscle relaxation, simply tense a muscle group for 10 seconds, then release the tension and relax the muscle group for 10 seconds.

3. Meditation: Meditation is a technique that involves focusing on the present moment and cultivating a sense of calm and relaxation. Meditation can help to reduce stress and promote relaxation. To perform meditation, simply find a quiet place to sit, close your eyes, and focus on your breath.

4. Yoga: Yoga is a form of exercise that involves stretching and gentle movements. Yoga can help to reduce stress and tension in the body, improve circulation, and promote relaxation.

5. Acupuncture: Acupuncture is a technique that involves inserting thin needles into specific points on the body. Acupuncture can help to regulate the nervous system and promote relaxation.

In addition to these techniques, Shiatsu massage therapy can also be an effective treatment option for calming the nervous system. Shiatsu massage therapy involves applying pressure to specific points on the body, which can help to promote relaxation, reduce tension, and improve overall health and wellness. During Shiatsu massage therapy for calming the nervous system, the practitioner will focus on applying pressure to specific points on the body that are associated with relaxation and stress relief. These points may be located on the head, neck, shoulders, back, and feet.

Balancing energy flow

In Traditional Chinese Medicine (TCM), it is believed that the body is made up of a network of energy pathways called meridians. These meridians are responsible for the flow of energy throughout the body, and when the flow of energy is disrupted, it can lead to imbalances and health issues. Shiatsu massage therapy is a technique that can be used to balance the flow of energy in the body and promote overall health and wellness.

Shiatsu massage therapy involves applying pressure to specific points on the body, which can help to promote relaxation, relieve pain, and improve overall health and wellness. During Shiatsu massage therapy for balancing energy flow, the practitioner will focus on applying pressure to specific points on the body that are associated with the meridians and energy flow.

In TCM, each meridian is associated with specific organs and functions in the body. For example, the liver meridian is associated with the liver, while the stomach meridian is associated with digestion. By applying pressure to these meridians, Shiatsu massage therapy can help to improve the flow of energy and promote balance in the body.

In addition to Shiatsu massage therapy, there are also other techniques that can be used to balance the flow of energy in the body. These include:

1. Acupuncture: Acupuncture is a technique that involves inserting thin needles into specific points on the body. Acupuncture can help to regulate the flow of energy in the body and promote balance.

2. Herbal medicine: Herbal medicine is a form of treatment that involves using herbs and other natural substances to promote health and wellness. Herbal medicine can be used to support the flow of energy and promote balance in the body.

3. Tai Chi: Tai Chi is a form of exercise that involves slow, flowing movements. Tai Chi can help to improve the flow of energy in the body and promote balance.

4. Qigong: Qigong is a form of exercise that involves breathing techniques, meditation, and gentle movements. Qigong can help to improve the flow of energy in the body and promote balance.

Shiatsu for emotional well-being

Shiatsu massage therapy is a powerful tool for promoting emotional well-being. Shiatsu massage therapy involves applying pressure to specific points on the body, which can help to promote relaxation, reduce stress, and improve overall health and wellness. By targeting specific areas of the body associated with emotional regulation, Shiatsu massage therapy can be an effective treatment option for individuals looking to improve their emotional well-being.

One of the primary benefits of Shiatsu massage therapy for emotional well-being is stress reduction. Stress is a major contributor to emotional imbalances, and can lead to symptoms such as anxiety, depression, and insomnia. Shiatsu massage therapy can help to reduce stress by promoting relaxation, reducing tension in the muscles, and improving circulation. By reducing stress, Shiatsu massage therapy can help to improve emotional regulation and promote overall well-being.

Another benefit of Shiatsu massage therapy for emotional well-being is its ability to promote relaxation. Relaxation is a critical component of emotional regulation, and can help to reduce feelings of anxiety, tension, and overwhelm. Shiatsu massage therapy can help to promote relaxation by activating the parasympathetic nervous system, which is responsible for the "rest and digest" response in the body. By promoting relaxation, Shiatsu massage therapy can help to improve emotional well-being and promote a sense of calm.

In addition to stress reduction and relaxation, Shiatsu massage therapy can also be used to target specific emotional imbalances. Each point on the body in Shiatsu massage therapy is associated with specific emotions and emotional imbalances. For example, the liver meridian is associated with anger and frustration, while the heart meridian is associated with joy and love. By targeting specific points on the body, Shiatsu massage therapy can help to promote emotional balance and improve overall emotional well-being.

Shiatsu massage therapy can also be used to promote self-awareness and mindfulness. During Shiatsu massage therapy, the practitioner will often encourage the client to focus on their breath and become more present in their body. This mindfulness practice can help to reduce stress and promote emotional regulation, as well as promote overall well-being.

Chapter Seven

Shiatsu for Specific Populations

Shiatsu massage therapy is a versatile treatment option that can be adapted to meet the specific needs of different populations. Whether you are seeking Shiatsu massage therapy for chronic pain, stress relief, or emotional regulation, there are many ways in which this technique can be tailored to meet your individual needs. In this article, we will explore some of the ways in which Shiatsu massage therapy can be used to benefit specific populations.

1. Pregnant women: Shiatsu massage therapy can be a safe and effective treatment option for pregnant women. Shiatsu massage therapy can help to relieve common pregnancy-related discomforts such as back pain, headaches, and swelling. Additionally, Shiatsu massage therapy can help to promote relaxation and reduce stress, which can be beneficial for both the mother and the baby.

2. Athletes: Shiatsu massage therapy can be a helpful treatment option for athletes who are experiencing muscle soreness, fatigue, or injuries. Shiatsu massage therapy can help to improve circulation, reduce muscle tension, and promote healing. Additionally, Shiatsu massage therapy can be used to promote relaxation and reduce stress, which can be helpful for athletes who are training intensively.

3. Elderly individuals: Shiatsu massage therapy can be a gentle and effective treatment option for elderly individuals who are experiencing pain, stiffness, or limited mobility. Shiatsu massage therapy can help to improve

circulation, reduce pain and inflammation, and promote relaxation. Additionally, Shiatsu massage therapy can help to promote emotional well-being, which can be important for older adults who may be experiencing feelings of isolation or depression.

4. Children: Shiatsu massage therapy can be a helpful treatment option for children who are experiencing anxiety, hyperactivity, or sleep disturbances. Shiatsu massage therapy can help to promote relaxation, reduce stress, and improve overall well-being. Additionally, Shiatsu massage therapy can be a gentle and non-invasive treatment option for children who may be hesitant to receive other types of treatments.

5. Individuals with chronic pain: Shiatsu massage therapy can be a helpful treatment option for individuals who are experiencing chronic pain. Shiatsu massage therapy can help to reduce pain and inflammation, improve circulation, and promote relaxation. Additionally, Shiatsu massage therapy can be used to target specific areas of pain or discomfort, which can be beneficial for individuals who are seeking relief from a specific condition.

Pregnant women

Shiatsu massage therapy is a safe and effective treatment option for pregnant women. Pregnancy is a time of physical and emotional changes, and Shiatsu massage therapy can be a helpful tool for managing some of the discomforts associated with pregnancy. In this article, we will explore some of the ways in which Shiatsu massage therapy can be used to benefit pregnant women.

1. Pain relief: As the body changes during pregnancy, women may experience a variety of aches and pains. Shiatsu massage therapy can help to relieve pain and discomfort by targeting specific areas of the body.

Common areas of pain during pregnancy include the lower back, hips, and legs, and Shiatsu massage therapy can be used to alleviate these discomforts.

2. Improved circulation: Shiatsu massage therapy can help to improve circulation, which can be beneficial for both the mother and the baby. Improved circulation can help to reduce swelling, promote healing, and improve overall health and wellness.

3. Reduced stress: Pregnancy can be a stressful time, and stress can have a negative impact on both the mother and the baby. Shiatsu massage therapy can help to reduce stress by promoting relaxation and reducing tension in the muscles. By reducing stress, Shiatsu massage therapy can help to promote emotional well-being and improve overall health.

4. Eased labor and delivery: Regular Shiatsu massage therapy during pregnancy can help to prepare the body for labor and delivery. Shiatsu massage therapy can help to promote relaxation, reduce tension in the muscles, and improve circulation, which can all be helpful during labor and delivery.

5. Improved sleep: Many pregnant women experience difficulty sleeping due to discomfort, stress, or anxiety. Shiatsu massage therapy can help to promote relaxation and reduce stress, which can improve sleep quality during pregnancy.

It is important to note that pregnant women should always seek treatment from a qualified and licensed Shiatsu massage therapist who has experience working with pregnant women. The therapist should be familiar with the specific needs of pregnant women and be able to adapt their treatment techniques accordingly. Additionally, pregnant women should always consult with their healthcare provider before beginning any new treatment regimen.

Elderly individuals

Shiatsu massage therapy is a gentle and effective treatment option that can be beneficial for elderly individuals. As we age, our bodies may experience a variety of physical and emotional changes, and Shiatsu massage therapy can be a helpful tool for managing some of these changes. In this article, we will explore some of the ways in which Shiatsu massage therapy can be used to benefit elderly individuals.

1. Pain relief: As we age, we may experience aches and pains due to conditions such as arthritis or other chronic conditions. Shiatsu massage therapy can help to relieve pain by targeting specific areas of the body. By reducing pain, Shiatsu massage therapy can help to improve overall comfort and well-being.

2. Improved circulation: As we age, our circulation may become less efficient, which can lead to a variety of health issues. Shiatsu massage therapy can help to improve circulation by stimulating the flow of blood and lymphatic fluid. Improved circulation can help to promote healing, reduce inflammation, and improve overall health.

3. Reduced stress: As we age, we may experience stress due to changes in our health, relationships, or living situation. Shiatsu massage therapy can help to reduce stress by promoting relaxation and reducing tension in the muscles. By reducing stress, Shiatsu massage therapy can help to promote emotional well-being and improve overall health.

4. Improved mobility: As we age, we may experience a decline in mobility due to conditions such as arthritis or other chronic conditions. Shiatsu massage therapy can help to improve mobility by reducing pain and stiffness in the joints and muscles. By improving mobility, Shiatsu massage therapy can help to promote independence and improve overall quality of life.

5. Improved sleep: Many elderly individuals experience difficulty sleeping due to pain, stress, or anxiety. Shiatsu massage therapy can help to promote relaxation and reduce stress, which can improve sleep quality. By improving sleep quality, Shiatsu massage therapy can help to promote overall health and well-being.

It is important to note that elderly individuals should always seek treatment from a qualified and licensed Shiatsu massage therapist who has experience working with elderly clients. The therapist should be familiar with the specific needs of elderly individuals and be able to adapt their treatment techniques accordingly. Additionally, elderly individuals should always consult with their healthcare provider before beginning any new treatment regimen.

Athletes

Shiatsu massage therapy is a valuable treatment option for athletes looking to enhance their performance and recover from physical activity. Athletes often place significant physical demands on their bodies, which can lead to injuries and other health issues. Shiatsu massage therapy can help to prevent injuries, reduce pain, and improve overall athletic performance. In this article, we will explore some of the ways in which Shiatsu massage therapy can benefit athletes.

1. Injury prevention: Shiatsu massage therapy can help to prevent injuries by improving flexibility, reducing muscle tension, and promoting better body alignment. By maintaining good muscle health and flexibility, athletes can reduce their risk of injury during physical activity.

2. Improved circulation: Shiatsu massage therapy can help to improve circulation by stimulating blood flow and promoting the flow of lymphat-

ic fluid. Improved circulation can help to reduce inflammation, promote healing, and improve overall athletic performance.

3. Reduced pain: Shiatsu massage therapy can help to reduce pain by targeting specific areas of the body that may be causing discomfort. By reducing pain, athletes can train more effectively and improve their overall athletic performance.

4. Improved recovery: Shiatsu massage therapy can help to improve recovery after physical activity by reducing muscle soreness and promoting relaxation. By improving recovery, athletes can reduce their risk of injury and improve their overall athletic performance.

5. Improved focus: Shiatsu massage therapy can help to promote relaxation and reduce stress, which can improve focus and mental clarity. By improving focus, athletes can train more effectively and improve their overall athletic performance.

It is important to note that athletes should always seek treatment from a qualified and licensed Shiatsu massage therapist who has experience working with athletes. The therapist should be familiar with the specific needs of athletes and be able to adapt their treatment techniques accordingly. Additionally, athletes should always consult with their coach or healthcare provider before beginning any new treatment regimen.

Chapter Eight

Shiatsu for Prevention and Maintenance

Shiatsu massage therapy is not only a helpful tool for managing specific conditions or ailments, but it can also be used for prevention and maintenance. Regular Shiatsu massage therapy sessions can help to promote overall health and well-being by addressing imbalances in the body and promoting relaxation. In this article, we will explore some of the ways in which Shiatsu massage therapy can be used for prevention and maintenance.

1. Promoting relaxation: Shiatsu massage therapy can help to promote relaxation by reducing muscle tension and promoting deep breathing. By promoting relaxation, Shiatsu massage therapy can help to reduce stress and promote overall well-being.

2. Improving circulation: Shiatsu massage therapy can help to improve circulation by stimulating blood flow and promoting the flow of lymphatic fluid. Improved circulation can help to promote overall health and prevent conditions such as high blood pressure, varicose veins, and more.

3. Improving immune function: Shiatsu massage therapy can help to improve immune function by stimulating the flow of lymphatic fluid and promoting the elimination of toxins from the body. By improving immune function, Shiatsu massage therapy can help to prevent illness and promote overall health.

4. Improving digestion: Shiatsu massage therapy can help to improve digestion by promoting relaxation and reducing stress. By improving digestion, Shiatsu massage therapy can help to prevent digestive issues such as constipation, bloating, and more.

5. Improving sleep: Shiatsu massage therapy can help to improve sleep by promoting relaxation and reducing stress. By improving sleep quality, Shiatsu massage therapy can help to promote overall health and well-being.

It is important to note that Shiatsu massage therapy should not be used as a substitute for medical care or treatment. However, regular Shiatsu massage therapy sessions can be a helpful tool for promoting overall health and well-being. Shiatsu massage therapy should be performed by a qualified and licensed practitioner who can provide personalized treatment options tailored to your specific needs and concerns.

Boosting the immune system

The immune system is our body's defense mechanism against harmful pathogens and diseases. Keeping the immune system strong and healthy is essential for preventing illnesses and promoting overall well-being. Shiatsu massage therapy can be a helpful tool for boosting the immune system and promoting overall health. In this article, we will explore some of the ways in which Shiatsu massage therapy can boost the immune system.

1. Promoting relaxation: Shiatsu massage therapy can help to promote relaxation by reducing muscle tension and promoting deep breathing. By promoting relaxation, Shiatsu massage therapy can help to reduce stress and promote overall well-being. Stress can weaken the immune system, so reducing stress can help to boost immune function.

2. Improving circulation: Shiatsu massage therapy can help to improve circulation by stimulating blood flow and promoting the flow of lymphatic fluid. Improved circulation can help to promote the elimination of toxins from the body and improve immune function.

3. Stimulating lymphatic function: Shiatsu massage therapy can help to stimulate lymphatic function, which is essential for immune system health. The lymphatic system helps to remove waste and toxins from the body and transports white blood cells, which are essential for fighting infections.

4. Reducing inflammation: Shiatsu massage therapy can help to reduce inflammation, which is associated with many chronic diseases. By reducing inflammation, Shiatsu massage therapy can help to improve immune function and promote overall health.

5. Balancing the body's energy: Shiatsu massage therapy can help to balance the body's energy, which can improve immune function. When the body's energy is balanced, the immune system is better able to function properly and fight off infections.

It is important to note that Shiatsu massage therapy should not be used as a substitute for medical care or treatment. However, regular Shiatsu massage therapy sessions can be a helpful tool for promoting overall health and boosting the immune system. Shiatsu massage therapy should be performed by a qualified and licensed practitioner who can provide personalized treatment options tailored to your specific needs and concerns.

Improving flexibility and mobility

Flexibility and mobility are essential components of overall health and well-being. Improving flexibility and mobility can help to prevent injuries, reduce pain, and promote better posture. Shiatsu massage therapy can be a helpful tool for improving flexibility and mobility. In this article, we will explore some of the ways in which Shiatsu massage therapy can improve flexibility and mobility.

1. Reducing muscle tension: Shiatsu massage therapy can help to reduce muscle tension, which can improve flexibility and mobility. When muscles are tense, they are less flexible and more prone to injury. By reducing muscle tension, Shiatsu massage therapy can help to improve range of motion and prevent injuries.

2. Increasing circulation: Shiatsu massage therapy can help to increase circulation, which can improve flexibility and mobility. Improved circulation helps to deliver oxygen and nutrients to the muscles, which can improve their function and flexibility.

3. Promoting relaxation: Shiatsu massage therapy can help to promote relaxation, which can improve flexibility and mobility. When the body is relaxed, muscles are more pliable and flexible. By promoting relaxation, Shiatsu massage therapy can help to improve range of motion and reduce the risk of injuries.

4. Stretching and mobilizing the body: Shiatsu massage therapy can help to stretch and mobilize the body, which can improve flexibility and mobility. Shiatsu massage therapists use a variety of techniques to stretch and mobilize the body, including finger pressure, palm pressure, and stretching.

5. Improving posture: Shiatsu massage therapy can help to improve posture, which can improve flexibility and mobility. Poor posture can lead to muscle imbalances and reduce range of motion. By improving posture, Shiatsu massage therapy can help to improve range of motion and prevent injuries.

It is important to note that Shiatsu massage therapy should not be used as a substitute for medical care or treatment. However, regular Shiatsu massage therapy sessions can be a helpful tool for improving flexibility and mobility. Shiatsu massage therapy should be performed by a qualified and licensed practitioner who can provide personalized treatment options tailored to your specific needs and concerns.

Balancing energy flow for overall health

Shiatsu is a Japanese massage therapy that is based on the principles of Traditional Chinese Medicine. According to these principles, the body is made up of energy pathways known as meridians, which carry the flow of vital energy or "Ki". When the flow of Ki is disrupted or blocked, it can lead to physical and emotional imbalances and illnesses. Shiatsu massage therapy is designed to balance the flow of Ki, which can promote overall health and well-being. In this article, we will explore the concept of balancing energy flow for overall health and how Shiatsu massage therapy can help.

The concept of balancing energy flow is rooted in Traditional Chinese Medicine, which holds that the body is composed of energy pathways known as meridians. These meridians are believed to connect different organs and parts of the body, carrying the flow of vital energy or "Ki". When the flow of Ki is disrupted or blocked, it can lead to physical and emotional imbalances and illnesses.

Shiatsu massage therapy is designed to balance the flow of Ki by applying finger pressure, palm pressure, stretching, and other techniques to the body's meridians. By working on specific points along these meridians, Shiatsu massage therapists can help to release blockages and improve the flow of Ki. This can help to promote overall health and well-being by restoring the body's natural balance.

Balancing energy flow through Shiatsu massage therapy can have a variety of benefits for overall health. Some of the potential benefits of balancing energy flow through Shiatsu massage therapy include:

1. Reduced stress and anxiety: Shiatsu massage therapy can help to reduce stress and anxiety by promoting relaxation and improving the flow of Ki. By releasing tension and promoting relaxation, Shiatsu massage therapy can help to reduce the physical and emotional symptoms of stress and anxiety.

2. Improved immune function: Balancing energy flow through Shiatsu massage therapy can help to improve immune function by promoting the flow of Ki. When the flow of Ki is disrupted or blocked, it can weaken the immune system and make the body more susceptible to illness. By restoring the natural flow of Ki, Shiatsu massage therapy can help to improve immune function and reduce the risk of illness.

3. Increased energy and vitality: Balancing energy flow through Shiatsu massage therapy can help to increase energy and vitality by promoting the flow of Ki. When the flow of Ki is disrupted or blocked, it can lead to feelings of fatigue and lethargy. By restoring the natural flow of Ki, Shiatsu massage therapy can help to increase energy and vitality.

4. Reduced pain and inflammation: Shiatsu massage therapy can help to reduce pain and inflammation by improving the flow of Ki. When the flow of Ki is disrupted or blocked, it can lead to pain and inflammation in the affected area. By restoring the natural flow of Ki, Shiatsu massage therapy can help to reduce pain and inflammation.

5. Improved digestion: Balancing energy flow through Shiatsu massage therapy can help to improve digestion by promoting the flow of Ki. When the flow of Ki is disrupted or blocked, it can lead to digestive problems such as bloating, constipation, and diarrhea. By restoring the natural flow

of Ki, Shiatsu massage therapy can help to improve digestion and reduce these symptoms.

Chapter Nine

Developing a Personal Shiatsu Routine

Shiatsu massage therapy is a powerful tool for promoting overall health and well-being by balancing the flow of vital energy or "Ki". While receiving Shiatsu treatments from a licensed practitioner can be beneficial, developing a personal Shiatsu routine can help to maintain the benefits of the therapy between sessions. In this article, we will explore the steps to developing a personal Shiatsu routine.

1. Step 1: Identify your goals

The first step in developing a personal Shiatsu routine is to identify your goals. What do you hope to achieve through Shiatsu massage therapy? Are you looking to reduce stress and anxiety, improve immune function, increase energy and vitality, reduce pain and inflammation, or improve digestion? Identifying your goals can help to guide your personal Shiatsu routine.

2. Step 2: Learn the basic techniques

The next step is to learn the basic techniques of Shiatsu massage therapy. These include finger pressure, palm pressure, kneading, stretching, and other techniques that are designed to balance the flow of Ki. There are many resources available for learning these techniques, including books, videos, and online courses. It is important to learn these techniques properly to ensure that you are using them safely and effectively.

3. Step 3: Identify the meridians

The meridians are the energy pathways that run throughout the body, carrying the flow of Ki. Identifying the meridians that correspond to your goals can help to guide your personal Shiatsu routine. For example, if you are looking to reduce stress and anxiety, you may want to focus on the meridians that correspond to the heart and lungs.

4. Step 4: Create a routine

Once you have identified your goals, learned the basic techniques, and identified the meridians, you can create a personal Shiatsu routine. This may involve using specific techniques on certain points along the meridians that correspond to your goals. For example, if you are looking to reduce stress and anxiety, you may want to use finger pressure on the heart and lung meridians.

5. Step 5: Practice regularly

Consistency is key when it comes to developing a personal Shiatsu routine. It is important to practice regularly to maintain the benefits of the therapy. You may want to set aside a specific time each day to practice your routine, or incorporate it into your daily routine in other ways, such as during a break at work or before bed.

6. Step 6: Listen to your body

It is important to listen to your body when practicing Shiatsu massage therapy. If a particular technique or pressure point feels uncomfortable or painful, it may not be right for you. It is important to adjust your routine accordingly and consult with a licensed practitioner if you have any concerns.

Designing a sequence

Shiatsu massage therapy is a powerful healing modality that has been used for centuries to promote overall health and well-being. One of the key components of Shiatsu is designing a sequence of techniques that is tailored to the individual's specific needs and goals. In this article, we will explore the steps to designing a Shiatsu sequence.

1. Step 1: Assess the individual's needs

The first step in designing a Shiatsu sequencc is to assess the individual's needs. This may involve a consultation with the individual to discuss their goals, health history, and any specific concerns or areas of discomfort. The practitioner may also use traditional diagnostic techniques, such as pulse diagnosis or abdominal palpation, to further assess the individual's needs.

2. Step 2: Identify the meridians

Once the individual's needs have been assessed, the next step is to identify the meridians that correspond to those needs. Each meridian is associated with specific organs and functions in the body, and identifying the appropriate meridians is key to designing an effective sequence. For example, if the individual is experiencing digestive issues, the practitioner may focus on the stomach and spleen meridians.

3. Step 3: Choose the appropriate techniques

Once the meridians have been identified, the practitioner can choose the appropriate techniques to use in the sequence. These may include finger pressure, palm pressure, kneading, stretching, and other techniques. The specific techniques chosen will depend on the individual's needs and the meridians that are being targeted.

4. Step 4: Establish the order

Once the techniques have been chosen, the practitioner can establish the order in which they will be used in the sequence. This may involve starting with techniques that are more gentle and gradually increasing the pressure and intensity, or focusing on certain areas of the body before moving on to others. The order will depend on the individual's needs and the practitioner's expertise.

5. Step 5: Practice the sequence

Once the sequence has been established, the practitioner can begin practicing it on the individual. This may involve multiple sessions to refine and adjust the sequence as needed. It is important to listen to the individual's feedback and adjust the sequence accordingly to ensure that it is effective and comfortable for them.

6. Step 6: Provide guidance for at-home practice

In addition to practicing the sequence in the office, the practitioner may provide guidance for the individual to practice the sequence at home. This may involve providing diagrams or written instructions for the sequence, or guiding the individual through the sequence during the session to help them remember the techniques.

Tips for consistency and progression

Consistency and progression are essential components of any effective Shiatsu practice. Consistency involves regularly practicing Shiatsu techniques to maintain and improve their effectiveness over time, while progression involves gradually increasing the intensity and complexity of the techniques to achieve better results. In this article, we will explore some tips for achieving consistency and progression in your Shiatsu practice.

1. Tip 1: Establish a regular practice schedule

One of the most important tips for achieving consistency in your Shiatsu practice is to establish a regular practice schedule. This may involve setting aside a specific time each day or week to practice Shiatsu techniques, and sticking to that schedule as much as possible. By making Shiatsu a regular part of your routine, you are more likely to maintain consistency and see results over time.

2. Tip 2: Set goals and track progress

Another important tip for achieving consistency and progression in your Shiatsu practice is to set specific goals and track your progress over time. This may involve setting goals for specific meridians or areas of the body, or tracking your progress in terms of how you feel after each session. By setting goals and tracking your progress, you can stay motivated and monitor your progress over time.

3. Tip 3: Gradually increase the intensity and complexity of techniques

To achieve progression in your Shiatsu practice, it is important to gradually increase the intensity and complexity of the techniques you use. This may involve starting with more gentle techniques, such as finger pressure, and gradually incorporating more advanced techniques, such as stretching or kneading. By gradually increasing the intensity and complexity of your techniques, you can challenge your body and achieve better results over time.

4. Tip 4: Attend workshops and continuing education classes

Another important tip for achieving consistency and progression in your Shiatsu practice is to attend workshops and continuing education classes. These classes can provide you with new techniques and approaches to Shiatsu, as well as opportunities to practice and refine your skills. By continuing to learn and grow in your practice, you can maintain consistency and achieve greater results over time.

5. Tip 5: Practice self-care

Finally, it is important to practice self-care in your Shiatsu practice to maintain consistency and achieve progression. This may involve practicing techniques on yourself, receiving regular Shiatsu treatments from a licensed practitioner, and taking care of your overall health and well-being. By taking care of yourself, you can maintain consistency and achieve better results in your Shiatsu practice over time.

Integrating other wellness practices

Shiatsu is a powerful wellness practice that can be integrated with other wellness practices to create a holistic approach to health and well-being. By combining Shiatsu with other practices such as yoga, meditation, and nutrition, individuals can create a comprehensive approach to wellness that addresses the mind, body, and spirit. In this article, we will explore some ways in which Shiatsu can be integrated with other wellness practices to create a holistic approach to wellness.

Integrating Shiatsu with Yoga

Yoga and Shiatsu are both practices that focus on promoting balance and harmony within the body. By integrating Shiatsu with yoga, individuals can create a powerful wellness practice that addresses both the physical and energetic aspects of the body. Shiatsu can be used to release tension and promote relaxation in specific areas of the body, while yoga can be used to stretch and strengthen the entire body. Together, these practices can help to promote physical health, mental clarity, and spiritual growth.

Integrating Shiatsu with Meditation

Meditation is a practice that promotes mental clarity and inner peace. By integrating Shiatsu with meditation, individuals can create a powerful wellness practice that addresses both the physical and mental aspects of the body. Shiatsu can be used to release tension and promote relaxation in specific areas of the body, while meditation can be used to quiet the mind and promote inner peace. Together, these practices can help to promote overall well-being and reduce stress and anxiety.

Integrating Shiatsu with Nutrition

Nutrition is an important component of overall health and well-being. By integrating Shiatsu with nutrition, individuals can create a comprehensive approach to wellness that addresses both the physical and nutritional needs of the body. Shiatsu can be used to promote relaxation and improve digestion, while nutrition can be used to provide the body with the nutrients it needs to function at its best. Together, these practices can help to promote overall health and vitality.

Integrating Shiatsu with Acupuncture

Acupuncture is a practice that uses thin needles to stimulate specific points on the body to promote healing and balance. By integrating Shiatsu with acupuncture, individuals can create a powerful wellness practice that addresses both the physical and energetic aspects of the body. Shiatsu can be used to promote relaxation and improve circulation, while acupuncture can be used to stimulate specific points on the body to promote healing and balance. Together, these practices can help to promote overall health and well-being.

Integrating Shiatsu with Mindfulness

Mindfulness is a practice that involves being present in the moment and paying attention to one's thoughts, feelings, and surroundings. By integrating Shiatsu with mindfulness, individuals can create a powerful wellness practice that addresses both the physical and mental aspects of the body. Shiatsu can be used to promote relaxation and improve circulation, while mindfulness can be used to promote mental clarity and reduce stress and anxiety. Together, these practices can help to promote overall health and well-being.

Chapter Ten

Becoming a Shiatsu Practitioner

Shiatsu is a unique form of bodywork that originated in Japan and has gained popularity worldwide for its holistic approach to healing. As a result, many individuals have become interested in becoming a Shiatsu practitioner themselves. Below we will explore the various aspects of becoming a Shiatsu practitioner, including education, training, and certification.

One of the first steps to becoming a Shiatsu practitioner is to gain a solid understanding of the principles and philosophy of Shiatsu. This includes knowledge of the meridian system, the concept of Ki, and the techniques used in Shiatsu. It is important to have a thorough understanding of the principles of Shiatsu before beginning any formal training.

Education and training programs for Shiatsu vary widely and are offered in many countries. In general, these programs cover the basic principles and techniques of Shiatsu, as well as the theory of Traditional Chinese Medicine (TCM) and anatomy and physiology. Many programs also require students to complete a certain number of hours of clinical practice to gain hands-on experience.

One of the key aspects of becoming a Shiatsu practitioner is learning how to properly apply finger pressure, palm pressure, kneading, and stretching techniques to the body. These techniques are used to stimulate the meridian system and balance the flow of Ki throughout the body. Learning proper body mechanics is also crucial for preventing injury and ensuring the safety of both the practitioner and the client.

In addition to technical skills, it is important for Shiatsu practitioners to develop effective communication and listening skills to understand their clients' needs and provide personalized treatment. The ability to establish a comfortable and safe environment for clients is also essential for building trust and fostering healing.

Certification and licensing requirements for Shiatsu practitioners vary by country and region. In some places, there are no formal requirements, while in others, practitioners must complete a certain number of training hours and pass an exam to become licensed. It is important to research the specific requirements in your area before pursuing a career as a Shiatsu practitioner.

Once certified, Shiatsu practitioners may choose to work in a variety of settings, including private practices, wellness centers, spas, and hospitals. Some practitioners may also choose to specialize in working with specific populations, such as athletes, pregnant women, or the elderly.

To become a successful Shiatsu practitioner, it is important to continue learning and expanding your knowledge and skills. This may include attending workshops, continuing education courses, and staying up to date with the latest research in the field.

Training and certification

Shiatsu is a Japanese massage technique that uses finger pressure and other massage techniques to promote physical and emotional well-being. While anyone can practice basic Shiatsu techniques at home, becoming a professional Shiatsu practitioner requires specialized training and certification.

Training and certification requirements for Shiatsu practitioners can vary depending on the country and region. In Japan, for example, Shiatsu is recognized as a licensed medical practice and requires a minimum of 2,500 hours of training. In other countries, such as the United States, certification may not be required, but practitioners may choose to pursue training and certification through private Shiatsu schools or organizations.

Training in Shiatsu typically involves a combination of classroom instruction, hands-on practice, and supervised clinical experience. Coursework may cover topics such as anatomy, physiology, traditional Chinese medicine, and the principles and techniques of Shiatsu. Students will also practice various Shiatsu techniques, such as finger pressure, palm pressure, and stretching, on classmates and clients under the guidance of experienced instructors.

In addition to coursework, many Shiatsu training programs require students to complete a certain number of supervised clinical hours. During these hours, students work with real clients to practice their techniques and gain hands-on experience in a supervised setting.

After completing the required training and clinical hours, aspiring Shiatsu practitioners may choose to pursue certification through a professional organization or school. Certification may involve passing a written exam, demonstrating proficiency in various Shiatsu techniques, and completing a certain number of continuing education hours each year.

In addition to formal training and certification, successful Shiatsu practitioners should possess certain personal and professional qualities. Strong communication skills are essential, as practitioners must be able to listen to clients' concerns and communicate effectively with them about their treatment plans. Patience, compassion, and a strong desire to help others are also important qualities for Shiatsu practitioners.

1. Shiatsu practitioners may work in a variety of settings, such as private practices, spas, or wellness centers. Some practitioners may choose to specialize in certain areas, such as working with pregnant women or athletes. Regardless of their specialty, all Shiatsu practitioners share a common goal: to help clients achieve physical and emotional balance and well-being through the power of touch.

Ethics and professional standards

Shiatsu, like any other holistic practice, has its own set of ethical and professional standards that practitioners are expected to adhere to. These standards ensure that clients receive safe and effective treatments and that practitioners maintain a high level of professionalism and integrity.

One of the primary ethical standards for Shiatsu practitioners is informed consent. Practitioners must ensure that their clients are fully informed about the nature of the treatment, including its benefits and potential risks. They should also provide clients with a clear explanation of the treatment plan and any alternative options. Informed consent also includes obtaining permission from clients before performing any new techniques or procedures.

Another ethical standard is maintaining client confidentiality. Practitioners must ensure that any personal or medical information shared by their clients is kept confidential and not disclosed to third parties without the client's consent. This confidentiality also extends to maintaining secure records of client information.

Professional standards require Shiatsu practitioners to maintain a high level of competence and ongoing professional development. This includes maintaining knowledge of the latest techniques and research in the field and continuously improving their skills through ongoing education and training. Practitioners should also be aware of their own limitations and seek advice or refer clients to other professionals when appropriate.

Practitioners must also maintain appropriate boundaries and professional conduct with clients. They should avoid any behavior that could be perceived as inappropriate, such as engaging in personal relationships with clients, providing treatments in non-professional settings, or using their position to exploit clients in any way.

Another important aspect of ethical and professional standards in Shiatsu is ensuring that practitioners are properly trained and certified. Practitioners should receive training from reputable institutions and obtain appropriate certification from recognized governing bodies. This helps ensure that practitioners are competent, knowledgeable, and practicing within a recognized code of conduct.

In addition to these ethical and professional standards, there are also legal and regulatory requirements that Shiatsu practitioners must adhere to. This includes obtaining any necessary permits or licenses, following health and safety regulations, and adhering to any local or national laws related to the practice of Shiatsu.

Building a successful practice

Shiatsu is a powerful form of bodywork that can help clients with a wide range of physical, emotional, and mental health issues. As a Shiatsu practitioner, building a successful practice requires a combination of technical skills, communication skills, and business acumen. Below we will we'll explore some of the key considerations for building a successful Shiatsu practice.

The first step in building a successful Shiatsu practice is to develop your technical skills. This involves completing a comprehensive Shiatsu training program that covers the essential principles and techniques of this modality. While there are many training programs available, it's important to choose one that is recognized by a reputable Shiatsu organization, such as the Shiatsu Society in the UK or the American Organization for Bodywork Therapies of Asia in the US.

Once you have completed your training, it's important to continue developing your skills through ongoing education and professional development. This can involve attending workshops, seminars, and conferences to learn new techniques, deepen your understanding of the body, and stay up-to-date with the latest research and trends in the field.

In addition to technical skills, communication skills are also essential for building a successful Shiatsu practice. Effective communication involves being able to listen actively to your clients, understand their needs and concerns, and explain the benefits of Shiatsu in a clear and concise manner. This can help build trust and establish a strong therapeutic relationship with your clients, which can lead to increased satisfaction and repeat business.

To build your communication skills, it's important to practice active listening, ask open-ended questions, and provide clear and concise explanations of the Shiatsu process. You may also want to consider taking courses or workshops in communication skills or seeking the advice of a business coach or mentor who can help you develop these skills.

In addition to technical and communication skills, building a successful Shiatsu practice also requires strong business acumen. This involves developing a business plan, setting goals, and implementing effective marketing strategies to attract and retain clients.

When developing your business plan, it's important to consider factors such as your target market, competition, pricing, and revenue projections. You may also want to consider factors such as insurance and liability coverage, office space, and equipment.

Marketing your Shiatsu practice can involve a variety of strategies, including networking, referrals, online marketing, and traditional advertising. It's important to choose marketing strategies that are effective for your target market and align with your personal values and brand.

Finally, it's important to maintain high ethical and professional standards in your Shiatsu practice. This involves adhering to a code of ethics and conduct, maintaining appropriate boundaries with clients, and ensuring confidentiality and privacy at all times.

To maintain ethical and professional standards, it's important to stay up-to-date with the latest research and trends in the field, seek the advice of colleagues and mentors, and participate in ongoing professional development and training opportunities.

Chapter Eleven

Shiatsu for Specific Conditions

Shiatsu is a traditional Japanese therapy that has been practiced for centuries. It is based on the principles of traditional Chinese medicine and uses finger pressure, stretching, and other techniques to balance the body's energy flow and promote healing. Shiatsu is a holistic therapy that can be used to address a wide range of physical and emotional conditions. Below we will discuss some specific conditions that can be treated with Shiatsu.

Anxiety and Depression

Shiatsu can be an effective therapy for anxiety and depression. It works by reducing stress and promoting relaxation. The therapist will use gentle finger pressure and stretching to help release tension in the body and promote a sense of calm. Regular Shiatsu sessions can help reduce symptoms of anxiety and depression over time.

Headaches and Migraines

Shiatsu can be an effective therapy for headaches and migraines. It works by reducing tension in the neck, shoulders, and head. The therapist will use finger pressure and stretching to help release tension in these areas, which can help alleviate headache pain. Regular Shiatsu sessions can help reduce the frequency and intensity of headaches and migraines.

Back Pain

Shiatsu can be an effective therapy for back pain. It works by reducing tension in the muscles and promoting circulation in the affected areas. The therapist will use finger pressure, stretching, and other techniques to help release tension and promote healing. Regular Shiatsu sessions can help reduce back pain and improve overall mobility.

Digestive Issues

Shiatsu can be an effective therapy for digestive issues. It works by promoting relaxation and reducing stress, which can help improve digestion. The therapist will use finger pressure and stretching to help stimulate the digestive system and promote healthy digestion. Regular Shiatsu sessions can help alleviate symptoms of digestive issues such as bloating, constipation, and acid reflux.

Insomnia

Shiatsu can be an effective therapy for insomnia. It works by reducing stress and promoting relaxation, which can help improve sleep quality. The therapist will use finger pressure and stretching to help release tension in the body and promote a sense of calm. Regular Shiatsu sessions can help improve sleep quality and reduce the frequency of insomnia.

Menstrual Issues

Shiatsu can be an effective therapy for menstrual issues such as cramps, irregular periods, and PMS. It works by promoting circulation and reducing tension in the muscles and organs of the reproductive system. The therapist will use finger pressure and stretching to help promote healthy circulation and alleviate symptoms of menstrual issues. Regular Shiatsu sessions can help reduce the severity and frequency of menstrual issues.

Respiratory Issues

Shiatsu can be an effective therapy for respiratory issues such as asthma and allergies. It works by promoting relaxation and reducing tension in the muscles of the respiratory system. The therapist will use finger pressure and stretching to help promote healthy breathing and alleviate symptoms of respiratory issues. Regular Shiatsu sessions can help reduce the severity and frequency of respiratory issues.

Anxiety and depression

Anxiety and depression are two common mental health conditions that affect millions of people around the world. They can be caused by a variety of factors, such as genetic predisposition, traumatic life events, chronic stress, and more. While there are many treatment options available, including medication and talk therapy, an increasing number of individuals are turning to alternative and complementary therapies, such as Shiatsu, to manage their symptoms.

Shiatsu, a Japanese form of bodywork, is based on the principles of Traditional Chinese Medicine (TCM), which views the body as a whole and emphasizes the importance of maintaining balance and harmony between the various systems and organs. According to TCM, anxiety and depression are often caused by imbalances or blockages in the flow of energy, or Qi, throughout the body. By stimulating certain acupressure points and meridians, Shiatsu practitioners aim to release tension and promote the free flow of Qi, which can lead to a greater sense of calm and relaxation.

There are several Shiatsu techniques that can be used to address anxiety and depression, including:

1. Finger pressure: This involves applying firm pressure to specific points on the body using the fingers, thumbs, or knuckles. Some of the points that may be targeted for anxiety and depression include the Bai Hui point

on the top of the head, the Shen Men point on the ear, and the Yin Tang point between the eyebrows.

2. Palm pressure: This involves using the palms of the hands to apply gentle pressure to the body, such as the back or the shoulders. This can help to release tension and promote relaxation.

3. Stretching: This involves gently stretching the body to release tension and increase flexibility. This can be particularly helpful for individuals who carry a lot of tension in their muscles and may benefit from the release of physical tension.

4. Breathing techniques: This involves teaching clients deep breathing exercises to help them relax and manage their anxiety. This can be done both during a Shiatsu session and as a home practice.

5. Shiatsu massage: This involves using a combination of techniques, including finger pressure, palm pressure, and stretching, to promote relaxation and release tension in the body.

While Shiatsu can be a helpful tool for managing anxiety and depression, it is important to note that it should not be used as a substitute for medical treatment. Individuals who are experiencing severe or chronic symptoms should seek the advice of a healthcare professional and should not rely solely on Shiatsu or other alternative therapies. Additionally, Shiatsu practitioners should work in conjunction with other healthcare providers to ensure that clients are receiving comprehensive care.

In addition to Shiatsu, there are other complementary therapies that may be helpful for managing anxiety and depression, such as acupuncture, mindfulness meditation, and yoga. These practices can also help to promote relaxation and reduce stress, and may be used in conjunction with Shiatsu to provide a more holistic approach to healing.

Chronic pain management

Chronic pain is a widespread condition that affects millions of people worldwide. It can significantly affect one's quality of life, making it challenging to perform daily tasks and engage in physical activities. While there are various treatment options for chronic pain, such as medication and physical therapy, Shiatsu massage has been gaining recognition as an effective form of therapy for pain management.

Shiatsu massage is a Japanese form of massage that uses finger pressure on specific points of the body to stimulate the body's natural healing process. It is based on the principles of Traditional Chinese Medicine and the concept of Qi, which is the vital energy that flows through the body. Shiatsu massage aims to balance the flow of Qi to promote overall health and wellness.

Chronic pain is often the result of imbalances in the body's Qi or energy flow. Shiatsu massage can help to restore balance and improve energy flow, which can reduce pain and discomfort. By applying pressure to specific points on the body, the massage therapist can stimulate the body's natural healing process, which can help to reduce inflammation and promote relaxation.

Shiatsu massage can be beneficial for various types of chronic pain, including back pain, neck pain, shoulder pain, and joint pain. It can also be helpful for conditions such as fibromyalgia, arthritis, and migraines. The massage therapist will typically begin by assessing the patient's pain levels and determining the best approach for their specific needs.

During a Shiatsu massage session, the patient lies down on a massage table, fully clothed. The therapist will use their fingers, palms, and thumbs to apply pressure to specific points on the body, known as acupressure points.

The pressure is typically deep and sustained, and the therapist may also use stretching and other techniques to help release tension in the muscles and promote relaxation.

One of the benefits of Shiatsu massage for chronic pain management is that it is a non-invasive form of therapy. Unlike medication or surgery, Shiatsu massage does not have any harmful side effects. It is a safe and natural way to manage pain and improve overall health and wellness.

Another benefit of Shiatsu massage is that it can be customized to the patient's individual needs. The massage therapist can adjust the pressure and intensity of the massage based on the patient's pain levels and preferences. They can also target specific areas of the body that are experiencing pain or tension.

In addition to Shiatsu massage, patients with chronic pain may also benefit from incorporating other forms of therapy into their treatment plan. For example, acupuncture, yoga, and meditation can all help to reduce pain and improve overall health and wellness. Patients should work with their healthcare providers to determine the best approach for their specific needs.

Supporting cancer care

Shiatsu is a traditional Japanese form of massage therapy that has been used for centuries to support the healing and well-being of individuals. In recent years, Shiatsu has gained increasing recognition as a complementary therapy for individuals receiving cancer treatment. Below we will explore the ways in which Shiatsu can support individuals receiving cancer care.

Cancer treatments such as chemotherapy and radiation can cause a range of physical and emotional side effects. Shiatsu can help alleviate these side effects and provide a sense of relaxation and well-being. Shiatsu works by applying pressure to specific points on the body, which helps to release tension and promote the body's natural healing processes. This can be particularly beneficial for individuals undergoing cancer treatment, as it can help manage symptoms such as pain, nausea, and fatigue.

One of the benefits of Shiatsu for individuals with cancer is its ability to help manage pain. Cancer treatments such as surgery, chemotherapy, and radiation can cause pain and discomfort. Shiatsu can help alleviate this pain by targeting specific points on the body that are associated with pain relief. By applying pressure to these points, Shiatsu can help release tension and promote the body's natural pain-relieving processes.

Shiatsu can also help manage nausea and other digestive issues that can be a side effect of cancer treatment. By applying pressure to specific points on the body, Shiatsu can help promote the flow of energy and relieve tension in the digestive system. This can help alleviate symptoms such as nausea, bloating, and constipation.

Fatigue is another common side effect of cancer treatment, and Shiatsu can help manage this symptom as well. By promoting relaxation and reducing tension in the body, Shiatsu can help restore energy levels and improve overall well-being. This can be particularly beneficial for individuals undergoing cancer treatment, as it can help them manage the physical and emotional demands of treatment.

In addition to managing physical symptoms, Shiatsu can also support emotional well-being for individuals with cancer. A cancer diagnosis can be overwhelming and stressful, and Shiatsu can help promote a sense of relaxation and calm. By reducing stress and tension in the body, Shiatsu can help individuals cope with the emotional challenges of cancer treatment and improve their overall quality of life.

It is important to note that Shiatsu is not a substitute for medical treatment, but rather a complementary therapy that can be used in conjunction with traditional cancer treatments. Before starting Shiatsu or any other complementary therapy, individuals should consult with their healthcare provider to ensure it is safe and appropriate for their specific condition.

Chapter Twelve

Self-Shiatsu Techniques

Self-Shiatsu is a practice of using Shiatsu massage techniques on oneself to promote relaxation, relieve tension, and alleviate pain. This practice can be a powerful tool for self-care and can be easily incorporated into daily routines. Below we will explore the benefits of self-Shiatsu and some techniques that can be practiced at home.

The benefits of self-Shiatsu are numerous. Firstly, it can help to reduce stress and tension in the body. The gentle pressure applied during self-Shiatsu can help to release tight muscles and calm the nervous system, promoting relaxation and a sense of calm. Secondly, it can help to alleviate pain and discomfort, especially in areas such as the neck, shoulders, and lower back. Regular practice of self-Shiatsu can improve blood and energy flow, which can lead to decreased inflammation and pain. Lastly, self-Shiatsu can help to improve overall health and well-being by supporting the body's natural healing processes.

There are various techniques that can be used for self-Shiatsu, depending on the area of the body that needs attention. Here are a few techniques that can be practiced at home:

1. Neck and shoulders: Begin by placing your right hand on your left shoulder and your left hand on your right shoulder. Apply gentle pressure with your fingers and thumbs and knead the muscles in a circular motion. Move your hands up and down along the sides of your neck, focusing on any areas of tension. Repeat on the other side.

2. Lower back: Sit comfortably with your feet flat on the floor. Place a tennis ball or massage ball under your lower back and lean against a wall or chair. Roll the ball up and down along your lower back, focusing on any areas of tension or pain.

3. Feet: Sit on a chair with your feet flat on the floor. Use your thumbs to apply pressure to the ball of your foot, moving in a circular motion. Move your thumbs along the arch and heel of your foot, focusing on any areas of tension. Repeat on the other foot.

4. Scalp: Sit comfortably and use your fingertips to gently massage your scalp in circular motions. Focus on any areas that feel tense or tight. This technique can help to alleviate headaches and promote relaxation.

It is important to practice self-Shiatsu with proper technique and care. Here are some tips to ensure safe and effective practice:

Start with gentle pressure and gradually increase as needed. Avoid applying too much pressure or force, as this can cause discomfort or injury.

Pay attention to your body's responses and adjust your technique accordingly. If a particular area feels too sensitive or painful, reduce the pressure or move to a different area.

Practice regularly for best results. Self-Shiatsu can be a helpful daily practice for promoting relaxation and reducing tension in the body.

Acupressure points for self-care

Acupressure is a traditional Chinese medicine practice that involves applying pressure to specific points on the body to stimulate the body's natural healing processes. Acupressure is often used as a form of self-care, and many people find it to be an effective way to alleviate pain, reduce stress, and promote overall well-being. Below we will discuss acupressure points for self-care and their benefits.

One of the most commonly used acupressure points for self-care is the LI4 or Large Intestine 4. This point is located on the webbing between the thumb and the index finger. Stimulating this point is said to help alleviate pain, relieve headaches and reduce stress. Many people find it helpful to apply firm pressure to this point for several seconds, then release and repeat several times.

Another commonly used acupressure point for self-care is the GB20 or Gallbladder 20. This point is located at the base of the skull, in the hollows on either side of the spine. Stimulating this point is said to help alleviate neck pain, headaches, and stress. To stimulate this point, use your thumbs to apply firm pressure to the area for several seconds, then release and repeat several times.

The PC6 or Pericardium 6 is another acupressure point commonly used for self-care. This point is located on the inner forearm, approximately two finger-widths above the wrist crease. Stimulating this point is said to help alleviate nausea, anxiety, and stress. To stimulate this point, use your index and middle fingers to apply firm pressure to the area for several seconds, then release and repeat several times.

The SP6 or Spleen 6 is another acupressure point commonly used for self-care. This point is located on the inner lower leg, approximately four finger-widths above the ankle bone. Stimulating this point is said to help alleviate menstrual cramps, digestive issues, and stress. To stimulate this point, use your index and middle fingers to apply firm pressure to the area for several seconds, then release and repeat several times.

In addition to these acupressure points, there are many other points on the body that can be stimulated to promote self-care and well-being. These points can be found in various locations throughout the body, and each point is associated with specific benefits and functions.

When practicing acupressure for self-care, it is important to use gentle pressure and to listen to your body's responses. If you experience discomfort or pain while stimulating a point, stop and move on to a different point or adjust your pressure. Additionally, it is important to consult with a healthcare provider before using acupressure as a form of self-care, especially if you have any underlying health conditions or concerns.

Daily routine for stress relief

Daily routine for stress relief with Shiatsu

Stress is a common problem that can affect anyone at any time. It can lead to a range of physical and mental health issues, such as anxiety, depression, and high blood pressure. While there are many ways to manage stress, Shiatsu is a holistic therapy that can help promote relaxation and balance in the body. Below we will explore a daily routine for stress relief with Shiatsu.

Shiatsu is a form of massage therapy that originated in Japan. It is based on the principles of Traditional Chinese Medicine (TCM) and uses finger pressure, palm pressure, and stretching techniques to balance the body's energy flow. The aim of Shiatsu is to promote relaxation, relieve tension, and improve overall wellbeing.

To incorporate Shiatsu into your daily routine for stress relief, you can follow these simple steps:

1. Step 1: Start with deep breathing

Deep breathing is a simple yet effective way to calm the mind and relax the body. Start by finding a quiet space where you can sit comfortably.

Close your eyes and take a deep breath in through your nose, hold for a few seconds, and then exhale slowly through your mouth. Repeat this for a few minutes, focusing on the sensation of the breath moving in and out of your body.

2. Step 2: Warm up with self-massage

Before starting any Shiatsu techniques, it's essential to warm up the body. Start by gently massaging your hands, wrists, and forearms using circular motions. Then move on to your neck and shoulders, using your fingers and thumbs to apply pressure and release any tension. Finally, use your palms to massage your lower back and hips.

3. Step 3: Focus on acupressure points

Acupressure points are specific points on the body that are believed to be connected to the body's energy meridians. By applying pressure to these points, you can help promote relaxation and balance in the body. Here are a few acupressure points that can help with stress relief:

4. The third eye point: Located between the eyebrows, this point is believed to help calm the mind and relieve stress.

5. The heart point: Located on the palm of the hand, in the center of the wrist, this point is believed to help promote relaxation and calmness.

6. The pericardium point: Located on the inner side of the forearm, about two inches above the wrist, this point is believed to help relieve stress and anxiety.

7. The bladder point: Located on the back of the neck, just below the hairline, this point is believed to help relieve tension and promote relaxation.

Apply gentle pressure to these points using your fingers or thumbs for a few minutes each.

8. Step 4: Use stretching techniques

Stretching is an essential part of Shiatsu and can help relieve tension in the muscles and improve flexibility. Here are a few simple stretching techniques you can try:

9. Shoulder stretch: Stand with your feet shoulder-width apart and your arms by your sides. Raise your shoulders up towards your ears, hold for a few seconds, and then release.

10. Neck stretch: Sit with your back straight and your shoulders relaxed. Tilt your head to the left, bringing your left ear towards your left shoulder. Hold for a few seconds, and then repeat on the right side.

11. Hamstring stretch: Sit on the floor with your legs straight out in front of you. Slowly lean forward, reaching towards your toes. Hold for a few seconds, and then release.

12. Step 5: End with relaxation

Finish your daily routine with a few minutes of relaxation. Lie down on your back, close your eyes, and focus on your breath. Visualize a peaceful place or imagine a calming color, such as blue or green. Stay in this

Shiatsu for neck and shoulder tension

Shiatsu massage is a traditional Japanese technique used to relieve physical and emotional tension by applying pressure to specific points on the body. Shiatsu is an excellent therapy for people who experience neck and shoulder tension due to stress, poor posture, or repetitive strain.

The neck and shoulder region is a common area of tension in the body, and stress often plays a role in causing this discomfort. People may experience tension headaches, muscle stiffness, and even limited range of motion as a result of neck and shoulder tension. Shiatsu massage can help to release this tension and promote relaxation, allowing individuals to experience relief from their symptoms.

Shiatsu practitioners focus on specific points along the meridian channels in the body that are associated with the neck and shoulder region. By applying pressure to these points, the practitioner can stimulate the flow of energy and promote healing in the affected area.

One of the primary meridians targeted during Shiatsu therapy for neck and shoulder tension is the Gallbladder meridian. This meridian runs along the side of the body, from the eye down to the fourth toe, and it is associated with the muscles and tendons of the neck and shoulder region. By applying pressure to specific points along this meridian, the practitioner can help to relieve tension and promote relaxation in the neck and shoulders.

In addition to targeting the Gallbladder meridian, Shiatsu practitioners may also focus on other meridians that can help to alleviate neck and shoulder tension. The Small Intestine meridian, for example, runs along the back of the arm and is associated with the trapezius muscle, which is often a source of tension in the shoulders. The Large Intestine meridian, which runs along the back of the arm and over the shoulder, is also targeted in Shiatsu therapy for neck and shoulder tension.

Shiatsu massage techniques for the neck and shoulders can include finger pressure, palm pressure, and kneading. Practitioners may also use stretching and rotation techniques to help increase range of motion and alleviate tension in the muscles and joints.

When performing Shiatsu for neck and shoulder tension, it is important for the practitioner to communicate with the client to ensure that the pressure is appropriate and comfortable. Clients should also be advised to communicate any discomfort or pain during the treatment to the practitioner, so that adjustments can be made as needed.

In addition to receiving Shiatsu therapy from a practitioner, individuals can also perform self-Shiatsu techniques to help relieve neck and shoulder tension. Acupressure points that can be targeted for self-care include the GB 20 points, located at the base of the skull, and the LI 4 points, located on the back of the hand between the thumb and index finger. Clients can use their fingers or thumbs to apply pressure to these points for several minutes at a time, several times a day.

Incorporating regular Shiatsu massage into a self-care routine can be an effective way to prevent and alleviate neck and shoulder tension. Daily stretches and exercises can also help to promote healthy posture and alleviate muscle stiffness in the neck and shoulders.

Chapter Thirteen

Shiatsu and Traditional Chinese Medicine (TCM)

Shiatsu is a traditional Japanese healing practice that has its roots in Traditional Chinese Medicine (TCM). TCM is a comprehensive system of healthcare that has been practiced in China for thousands of years. It is based on the concept of Qi, which is the vital energy that flows through the body. According to TCM, Qi flows through channels or pathways known as meridians. Shiatsu practitioners work with these meridians to help promote health and wellbeing.

TCM encompasses a variety of healing practices, including acupuncture, herbal medicine, and massage. Acupuncture involves the use of thin needles inserted into specific points along the meridians to stimulate the flow of Qi. Herbal medicine involves the use of herbs and other natural substances to promote health and treat illness. Massage, or Tui Na, involves the use of manual techniques to stimulate the flow of Qi and promote relaxation.

Shiatsu is a form of massage that incorporates many of the principles of TCM. Shiatsu practitioners use finger pressure, stretching, and other techniques to stimulate the flow of Qi and promote relaxation. Unlike traditional massage, which focuses on the muscles and soft tissues of the body, Shiatsu focuses on the meridians and energy flow.

In TCM, the meridians are associated with specific organs and functions of the body. For example, the lung meridian is associated with respiration, while the liver meridian is associated with the flow of Qi. Shiatsu practitioners work with these meridians to help promote health and treat illness.

Shiatsu is based on the concept of Ki, which is similar to the concept of Qi in TCM. Ki is the vital energy that flows through the body and is responsible for maintaining health and wellbeing. According to Shiatsu theory, when the flow of Ki is blocked or disrupted, it can lead to illness and other health problems. Shiatsu practitioners work to unblock and balance the flow of Ki to promote health and wellbeing.

Shiatsu practitioners use a variety of techniques to stimulate the flow of Ki and promote relaxation. Finger pressure is one of the most commonly used techniques in Shiatsu. Practitioners use their fingers, thumbs, and palms to apply pressure to specific points along the meridians. This pressure can help to unblock the flow of Ki and promote relaxation.

Another technique commonly used in Shiatsu is stretching. Shiatsu practitioners use stretching techniques to help loosen tight muscles and promote relaxation. They may also use techniques such as rocking or shaking to help release tension and promote relaxation.

In addition to finger pressure and stretching, Shiatsu practitioners may also use other techniques such as kneading or tapping. Kneading involves using the hands and fingers to apply pressure and massage the muscles. Tapping involves using the fingers to tap or drum on specific areas of the body to stimulate the flow of Ki and promote relaxation.

Shiatsu can be beneficial for a wide range of conditions, including chronic pain, stress, anxiety, and depression. It can also be helpful for promoting relaxation and improving overall wellbeing. Shiatsu is a gentle, non-invasive form of therapy that can be used in conjunction with other forms of healthcare to promote health and healing.

The five elements

Shiatsu, an ancient Japanese healing technique, is based on the principles of Traditional Chinese Medicine (TCM). One of the fundamental concepts in TCM is the Five Elements, which are a way of understanding the relationships between different aspects of nature and the human body. Below we will explore the Five Elements and their significance in Shiatsu.

The Five Elements, also known as the Five Phases or Five Movements, are Wood, Fire, Earth, Metal, and Water. Each element represents a specific energy, and they are related to different organs and body functions. The elements are also associated with emotions, seasons, colors, tastes, and other aspects of nature.

The Wood element represents growth and movement. It is associated with the liver and gallbladder organs and is related to the emotion of anger. The Fire element represents warmth, joy, and passion. It is associated with the heart and small intestine organs and is related to the emotion of joy. The Earth element represents stability and nourishment. It is associated with the spleen and stomach organs and is related to the emotion of worry. The Metal element represents strength and clarity. It is associated with the lung and large intestine organs and is related to the emotion of grief. The Water element represents fluidity and adaptability. It is associated with the kidney and bladder organs and is related to the emotion of fear.

In Shiatsu, the Five Elements are used to understand the client's physical, emotional, and energetic imbalances. Practitioners use various techniques to balance the client's energy flow and restore harmony to the affected element. For example, if a client presents with symptoms related to the Wood element, such as irritability or stiff joints, the practitioner may use techniques to release tension in the muscles and joints and improve the flow of energy to the liver and gallbladder.

Shiatsu practitioners may also use other TCM techniques, such as acupuncture or herbal medicine, to support the healing process. For example, an acupuncturist may use needles to stimulate specific points along the meridians associated with the affected element. Herbal medicine may be prescribed to support the organs and body functions related to the affected element.

In addition to its therapeutic benefits, Shiatsu can also provide insight into a client's overall well-being. The Five Elements can reveal patterns of imbalance that may indicate underlying emotional or mental stressors. For example, a client who presents with symptoms related to the Earth element, such as digestive issues or excessive worrying, may be experiencing stress related to work or personal relationships.

By addressing the root causes of these imbalances, Shiatsu can help clients achieve a greater sense of balance and overall well-being. Practitioners may also provide guidance on lifestyle changes, such as diet and exercise, to support the healing process.

Understanding yin and yang

Shiatsu is a Japanese bodywork therapy that is based on the principles of Traditional Chinese Medicine (TCM). TCM views the body as a whole, interconnected system that is in constant flux, with balance being the key to good health. Central to TCM is the concept of yin and yang, which are two complementary, yet opposing forces that govern the body's functions. Understanding yin and yang is essential for both the practitioner and the client in Shiatsu therapy.

According to TCM, everything in the universe, including the human body, is made up of yin and yang. Yin represents the passive, receptive, and feminine aspects, while yang represents the active, expansive, and masculine aspects. Yin and yang are not separate entities, but rather two parts of a whole that exist in dynamic balance. When this balance is disrupted, illness and disease can occur.

The theory of yin and yang can be applied to many aspects of the body, including the organs, tissues, and bodily functions. Each organ is classified as either yin or yang, and when they are in balance, they work together harmoniously to maintain health. For example, the heart is considered a yang organ because it pumps blood throughout the body, while the lungs are considered a yin organ because they receive and distribute oxygen to the body's tissues. When the heart and lungs are in balance, they support each other's functions and promote overall health.

1. In addition to the organs, yin and yang can also be applied to the bodily functions. TCM identifies five major bodily functions, each with its corresponding element: wood (liver), fire (heart), earth (spleen), metal (lung), and water (kidney). These elements are also associated with various yin and yang qualities, such as warmth, coolness, dryness, and moisture. In TCM, health is seen as the harmonious balance of these elements and their corresponding yin and yang qualities.

The principles of yin and yang can also be applied to the meridians, which are the energy pathways that run throughout the body. There are twelve primary meridians, each associated with a specific organ or bodily function. These meridians have both yin and yang aspects, and when they are in balance, the body's energy flows smoothly, promoting good health. However, when the energy is blocked or stagnant, it can lead to physical and emotional problems.

Shiatsu practitioners use their knowledge of yin and yang to identify imbalances in the body and help restore balance through various techniques, such as finger pressure, stretching, and manipulation of the body's energy flow. They may also recommend dietary and lifestyle changes to support the body's natural healing processes.

Integrating TCM concepts in shiatsu

Integrating Traditional Chinese Medicine (TCM) concepts in Shiatsu is an essential aspect of this Japanese massage therapy. The underlying principles of TCM and Shiatsu overlap in many ways and provide a holistic approach to healing the body, mind, and spirit. The integration of TCM concepts enhances the effectiveness of Shiatsu therapy, making it a unique and powerful healing modality.

TCM is a complete system of medicine that has been practiced for thousands of years in China. It is based on the belief that the body is a complex system of interconnected energy channels or meridians, and that a balance of yin and yang energies is essential for optimal health. TCM also recognizes the importance of the five elements - wood, fire, earth, metal, and water - in maintaining the balance of energy within the body.

Shiatsu, on the other hand, is a Japanese massage technique that uses finger pressure and other techniques to stimulate the body's energy flow. It is based on the principles of TCM and aims to balance the body's energy by releasing tension in the meridians. Shiatsu practitioners use their knowledge of the body's energy channels and points to provide deep relaxation, relieve pain, and promote healing.

One of the main TCM concepts integrated into Shiatsu is the concept of Qi, which refers to the body's vital energy. According to TCM, the body's Qi flows through meridians or channels, and blockages in these channels can cause pain, illness, and disease. Shiatsu practitioners use finger pressure on specific points on the body to release these blockages and restore the flow of Qi, promoting healing and well-being.

Another TCM concept that is integrated into Shiatsu is the concept of the five elements. Each element is associated with specific meridians, organs, emotions, and qualities. For example, the wood element is associated with the liver and gallbladder meridians, the emotion of anger, and the qualities of growth and creativity. Shiatsu practitioners use this knowledge to tailor the treatment to the individual's specific needs, addressing any imbalances in the body's energy flow.

The concept of yin and yang is also an essential aspect of TCM and Shiatsu. Yin and yang are opposing forces that are present in everything in the universe, including the body. Yin represents the feminine, passive, and cool energy, while yang represents the masculine, active, and warm energy. In TCM, an imbalance in yin and yang can cause illness and disease. Shiatsu practitioners aim to balance these opposing forces by using pressure on specific points on the body, promoting a sense of harmony and well-being.

Integrating TCM concepts into Shiatsu enhances the effectiveness of this therapy in many ways. Firstly, it provides a holistic approach to healing the body, mind, and spirit. Shiatsu practitioners can use their knowledge of TCM to address physical, emotional, and mental imbalances in the body, promoting overall well-being. Secondly, it allows for a personalized approach to treatment, tailoring the therapy to the individual's specific needs and imbalances. This approach recognizes that each person's body is unique and requires a personalized treatment plan.

Chapter Fourteen

Shiatsu and Western Medicine

Shiatsu is a form of manual therapy that originated in Japan and has gained popularity worldwide. It involves the use of finger pressure, stretching, and other techniques to balance the body's energy flow and promote health and well-being. While traditional Shiatsu is rooted in Eastern medicine, Western medicine has also taken an interest in this therapeutic technique. Below we will explore the integration of Shiatsu and Western medicine, including the benefits and challenges of combining these two approaches.

Western medicine is a system of healthcare that is based on scientific evidence and focuses on the diagnosis and treatment of specific illnesses or diseases. This approach relies on medical tests, medications, and surgical interventions to alleviate symptoms and cure the underlying condition. In contrast, Shiatsu is based on the principles of traditional Chinese medicine, which views the body as a whole and seeks to balance the flow of energy or Qi within it. Shiatsu therapists use their hands to apply pressure to specific points on the body, stimulating the nervous system and promoting relaxation, circulation, and healing.

Despite these differences, there are areas of overlap between Shiatsu and Western medicine. For example, both approaches recognize the importance of physical activity, diet, and stress reduction for maintaining good health. Additionally, many Western medical practitioners are beginning to recognize the benefits of complementary and alternative therapies like Shiatsu.

One of the main benefits of integrating Shiatsu and Western medicine is the potential for more holistic and personalized healthcare. By incorporating Shiatsu into their practice, Western medical practitioners can offer patients a more comprehensive approach to healing that addresses not only physical symptoms but also emotional and spiritual well-being. This can lead to improved patient outcomes, as patients who receive more personalized care are often more engaged in their own healing process and more likely to follow through with treatment plans.

Another potential benefit of integrating Shiatsu and Western medicine is the ability to reduce reliance on pharmaceuticals and other invasive treatments. Shiatsu can help manage a variety of conditions, including chronic pain, anxiety, and depression, without the need for medication or surgery. This can be particularly beneficial for patients who are wary of or unable to tolerate traditional medical interventions.

Despite these potential benefits, there are also challenges to integrating Shiatsu and Western medicine. One of the main challenges is the lack of scientific evidence supporting the efficacy of Shiatsu. While there is some research on the benefits of Shiatsu for certain conditions, such as chronic pain and anxiety, more studies are needed to establish its effectiveness and safety. This lack of evidence can make it difficult for Western medical practitioners to incorporate Shiatsu into their practice or to recommend it to their patients.

Another challenge is the need for more standardized training and certification for Shiatsu practitioners. Unlike Western medical practitioners, who undergo extensive education and training before practicing medicine, Shiatsu practitioners do not have a standardized certification process in many countries. This can make it difficult for patients to know whether a Shiatsu practitioner is qualified to provide safe and effective care.

Despite these challenges, the integration of Shiatsu and Western medicine has the potential to improve patient care and offer a more comprehensive approach to healing. More research is needed to establish the efficacy and safety of Shiatsu, and efforts should be made to establish standardized training and certification for Shiatsu practitioners. With these steps, the integration of Shiatsu and Western medicine can lead to better health outcomes and improved quality of life for patients.

Evidence-based research

Shiatsu is a form of Japanese bodywork that involves the application of pressure to specific points on the body. It is based on the principles of Traditional Chinese Medicine (TCM) and is believed to help balance the body's energy flow or Qi. While Shiatsu has been used for centuries to promote health and well-being, it has also been the subject of scientific research in recent years.

Research on Shiatsu has shown promising results in a variety of areas, including pain relief, stress reduction, and immune system enhancement. In a study published in the Journal of Alternative and Complementary Medicine, participants who received Shiatsu massage reported a significant reduction in pain and improved physical functioning compared to those who received a placebo treatment. Another study published in the International Journal of Neuroscience found that Shiatsu massage was effective in reducing stress levels and increasing feelings of relaxation.

Shiatsu has also been shown to have a positive effect on the immune system. A study published in the Journal of Psychosomatic Research found that Shiatsu massage increased the production of natural killer cells, which play an important role in the body's immune response. Another study published in the Journal of Alternative and Complementary Medicine found that Shiatsu massage was effective in improving sleep quality in individuals with insomnia.

While the evidence supporting Shiatsu is still somewhat limited, there is growing interest in the field of integrative medicine in using Shiatsu as a complementary therapy for a variety of health conditions. Many health-care providers are now integrating Shiatsu into their practices, and some insurance companies even cover the cost of Shiatsu treatments.

In addition to its potential health benefits, Shiatsu is also relatively safe and non-invasive. Unlike some other forms of bodywork, Shiatsu does not involve the use of oils or lotions and can be performed through clothing. It is generally well-tolerated by most individuals, although individuals with certain medical conditions, such as cancer or blood disorders, should consult with their healthcare provider before undergoing Shiatsu treatment.

Despite the growing interest in Shiatsu and its potential health benefits, more research is needed to fully understand its effects on the body. Future studies should focus on larger and more diverse populations, as well as the long-term effects of Shiatsu on various health outcomes.

Working with healthcare professionals

Shiatsu is a traditional Japanese bodywork therapy that has been used for centuries to promote relaxation, reduce stress, and alleviate pain. It involves the use of finger pressure, stretching, and other techniques to manipulate the body's energy flow and promote healing. In recent years, there has been an increased interest in the use of Shiatsu as a complementary therapy in healthcare settings. Below we will discuss how Shiatsu practitioners can work with healthcare professionals to promote wellness and improve patient outcomes.

Shiatsu is based on the principles of Traditional Chinese Medicine (TCM), which views the body as a complex system of interconnected energies. According to TCM, illness and disease occur when there is an imbalance or blockage in the flow of energy through the body. Shiatsu practitioners use finger pressure and other techniques to stimulate specific acupressure points on the body, which are believed to help restore balance and promote healing.

While Shiatsu is not a substitute for conventional medical treatment, it can be a valuable complement to other therapies. For example, Shiatsu has been shown to be effective in reducing pain and anxiety in cancer patients undergoing chemotherapy. In addition, it has been used to treat a variety of conditions, including back pain, headaches, digestive disorders, and sleep disorders.

To work effectively with healthcare professionals, Shiatsu practitioners need to understand the role of conventional medicine and the limitations of their own practice. They should be familiar with the common medical conditions and medications that their clients may be using, and should be able to communicate effectively with physicians and other healthcare providers.

One important area of collaboration between Shiatsu practitioners and healthcare professionals is in the management of chronic pain. Chronic pain is a complex condition that can be difficult to treat with conventional therapies. However, Shiatsu has been shown to be effective in reducing pain and improving quality of life in patients with chronic pain. By working together, Shiatsu practitioners and healthcare professionals can provide patients with a more comprehensive approach to pain management.

Another area of collaboration is in the treatment of mental health conditions. Shiatsu has been shown to be effective in reducing anxiety and depression, and can be used as a complementary therapy alongside conventional treatments such as medication and psychotherapy. By working with mental health professionals, Shiatsu practitioners can help patients manage their symptoms and improve their overall wellbeing.

In addition to working with healthcare professionals, Shiatsu practitioners can also collaborate with other complementary therapists to provide patients with a more holistic approach to healthcare. For example, Shiatsu can be combined with acupuncture, massage, and other bodywork therapies to provide a more comprehensive approach to pain management and wellness.

It is important for Shiatsu practitioners to maintain professional boundaries and recognize their limitations. While Shiatsu can be a valuable complement to other therapies, it is not a substitute for conventional medical treatment. Shiatsu practitioners should encourage their clients to seek medical advice when necessary and work collaboratively with healthcare professionals to ensure the best possible outcomes for their clients.

Integrating shiatsu into conventional treatments

Integrative medicine is becoming increasingly popular as more people seek out complementary therapies to supplement conventional treatments. One such therapy is Shiatsu, a form of Japanese massage that uses pressure points and stretches to improve overall health and well-being. Integrating Shiatsu into conventional treatments can be beneficial for patients in a variety of ways.

First, Shiatsu can help to alleviate physical symptoms and side effects of conventional treatments. For example, cancer patients undergoing chemotherapy often experience nausea, fatigue, and pain. Shiatsu can help to reduce these symptoms by promoting relaxation, increasing circulation, and stimulating the release of endorphins, the body's natural painkillers. Shiatsu can also help to improve the immune system, which is important for cancer patients whose immune systems are often weakened by chemotherapy.

Second, Shiatsu can provide emotional support for patients. Dealing with a chronic illness or serious health issue can be stressful and overwhelming, and many patients experience anxiety, depression, and other emotional difficulties. Shiatsu can help to reduce stress and promote relaxation, which can improve mood and overall emotional well-being. Shiatsu can also provide a sense of comfort and nurturing touch, which can be particularly beneficial for patients who may feel isolated or disconnected from others.

Third, Shiatsu can help to improve the overall effectiveness of conventional treatments. By promoting relaxation and reducing stress, Shiatsu can help to enhance the body's natural healing abilities. Shiatsu can also help to improve circulation and stimulate the lymphatic system, which can help to remove toxins from the body and improve overall health.

Integrating Shiatsu into conventional treatments requires communication and collaboration between healthcare professionals. Patients should inform their doctors and other healthcare providers that they are interested in receiving Shiatsu, and healthcare providers should be willing to discuss the benefits and risks of Shiatsu with their patients. Healthcare providers should also be willing to work with Shiatsu practitioners to develop a treatment plan that is safe and effective for their patients.

Shiatsu practitioners who are interested in integrating their practice into conventional healthcare settings should be knowledgeable about the benefits and risks of Shiatsu, as well as the specific needs and concerns of the patients they will be working with. They should also be willing to work collaboratively with healthcare providers, and should have a good understanding of the conventional treatments that their patients are receiving.

In order to ensure that Shiatsu is integrated into conventional treatments in a safe and effective manner, it is important to conduct research on the effectiveness of Shiatsu for specific health conditions. Evidence-based research can help to identify the most effective Shiatsu techniques for specific health conditions, as well as the potential risks and side effects of Shiatsu.

Integrating Shiatsu into conventional treatments can provide a number of benefits for patients, including alleviating physical symptoms, providing emotional support, and improving overall health and well-being. In order to ensure that Shiatsu is integrated into conventional treatments in a safe and effective manner, healthcare providers and Shiatsu practitioners should work collaboratively and be knowledgeable about the benefits and risks of Shiatsu. Evidence-based research can help to identify the most effective Shiatsu techniques for specific health conditions, and can help to ensure that Shiatsu is integrated into conventional treatments in a safe and effective manner.

Chapter Fifteen

Partner Shiatsu

Shiatsu is a form of therapeutic massage that has its roots in traditional Japanese medicine. While traditionally Shiatsu is performed by a practitioner on a client, partner Shiatsu is a practice that involves giving and receiving massage between two people. Below we will discuss partner Shiatsu, including its benefits, techniques, and how to get started.

Partner Shiatsu has many benefits, including stress relief, improved circulation, increased flexibility and mobility, and improved overall well-being. It can be a great way for couples, friends, or family members to connect with each other and improve their physical and emotional health. Partner Shiatsu is also a great way to learn more about Shiatsu and massage techniques in general.

There are many different techniques that can be used in partner Shiatsu, depending on the specific needs of the individuals involved. One technique is called shiatsu stretching, which involves using the hands and fingers to apply pressure to specific areas of the body while stretching the muscles. This technique is great for improving flexibility and mobility, and can be especially helpful for people who spend a lot of time sitting or standing in one position.

Another technique is called acupressure, which involves applying pressure to specific acupressure points on the body. These points are believed to correspond to specific organs and systems in the body, and applying pressure to these points can help improve overall health and well-being.

Acupressure can be particularly helpful for people experiencing pain or discomfort in specific areas of the body.

One important aspect of partner Shiatsu is communication. It's important for both partners to communicate their needs and preferences before, during, and after the massage. This can include things like which areas of the body need more attention, how much pressure to use, and what type of massage techniques to use. Clear communication can help ensure that both partners feel comfortable and that the massage is effective.

When getting started with partner Shiatsu, it's important to find a comfortable and quiet space where you can focus on the massage. You may want to use a mat or blanket to provide a comfortable surface for the massage. It's also important to have any necessary supplies on hand, such as massage oil or lotion.

To begin, start with a few minutes of deep breathing and relaxation exercises to help both partners relax and become more present. Then, begin with some basic massage techniques, such as gentle kneading or circular motions on the back, neck, and shoulders. From there, you can explore different techniques and areas of the body, depending on the needs and preferences of both partners.

Techniques for couples and friends

Shiatsu is a form of Japanese massage that can be used to promote relaxation, reduce stress, and improve overall well-being. While it is typically performed by a trained practitioner, shiatsu can also be used as a technique for couples and friends to use on each other.

When performing partner shiatsu, it is important to establish clear communication and boundaries. Both people should be comfortable with the level of pressure and the areas being worked on. It can be helpful to establish a code word or signal to indicate if the pressure is too much or if a break is needed.

There are several techniques that can be used for partner shiatsu. One of the simplest techniques is to use the thumbs to apply pressure to the base of the skull, working in circular motions. This can help to release tension in the neck and shoulders.

Another technique is to use the palm of the hand to apply pressure to the back, working in long strokes from the top of the shoulders to the lower back. This can help to improve circulation and reduce tension in the muscles.

A third technique is to use the knuckles to apply pressure to the hands and feet, working in circular motions. This can help to stimulate acupressure points and improve energy flow throughout the body.

Partner shiatsu can also involve stretches and joint mobilization. For example, one partner can gently stretch the other's arms and legs, using slow and controlled movements. This can help to improve flexibility and reduce stiffness in the joints.

Breathing techniques can also be incorporated into partner shiatsu. Both partners can focus on taking deep, slow breaths as pressure is applied. This can help to enhance relaxation and reduce stress.

It is important to keep in mind that partner shiatsu is not a substitute for professional massage therapy or medical treatment. If either partner has any underlying health conditions or concerns, they should consult with a healthcare provider before trying partner shiatsu.

Partner shiatsu can be a wonderful way for couples and friends to connect, relax, and support each other's health and well-being. By incorporating these simple techniques into your routine, you can experience the benefits of shiatsu from the comfort of your own home.

Effective communication during sessions

Effective communication is crucial for any successful shiatsu session. The practitioner must be able to establish a sense of trust and understanding with the client in order to create a safe and comfortable environment. Below we will explore various techniques for effective communication during shiatsu sessions.

First and foremost, active listening is a key component of effective communication. The practitioner should give their full attention to the client, both verbally and non-verbally. This means actively listening to the client's concerns and being attentive to their body language, tone of voice, and other nonverbal cues. By doing so, the practitioner can establish a deeper connection with the client and gain a better understanding of their needs.

Another important aspect of effective communication during a shiatsu session is using clear and concise language. The practitioner should avoid using medical jargon or technical terms that the client may not understand. Instead, they should use simple and clear language to explain the techniques being used and their benefits. This not only helps the client understand the treatment, but also puts them at ease.

Body language is also an essential aspect of effective communication during a shiatsu session. The practitioner should be aware of their own body language and how it may affect the client. For example, crossing one's arms or appearing closed off can create a sense of distance and mistrust. On the other hand, maintaining an open and welcoming posture can help the client feel more at ease and encourage them to communicate openly.

During the session, it's important for the practitioner to check in with the client regularly to ensure their comfort and safety. This can be done by asking simple questions, such as "Is this pressure okay?" or "How are you feeling?" These check-ins can also provide an opportunity for the client to communicate any concerns or discomfort they may be experiencing.

It's also important for the practitioner to respect the client's boundaries and preferences. This means asking for consent before beginning any techniques and ensuring the client is comfortable with the level of pressure being used. If the client expresses discomfort or requests a change in technique, the practitioner should adjust accordingly.

Finally, effective communication during a shiatsu session also involves setting clear expectations and boundaries from the outset. The practitioner should explain the purpose and goals of the session, as well as any limitations or contraindications. This helps to establish a clear understanding of what will happen during the session and what the client can expect.

Adapting pressure and technique

Shiatsu is a traditional Japanese massage technique that involves the application of pressure to specific points on the body to promote healing and relaxation. While it is a relatively gentle technique, it can be adapted to suit the needs of each individual client. One important aspect of adapting shiatsu to different clients is adjusting the pressure and technique used during the massage.

The pressure used during shiatsu can vary greatly depending on the needs and preferences of the client. Some people may prefer deeper pressure to release tension and tightness, while others may be more sensitive and require a lighter touch. It is important for the practitioner to communicate with the client throughout the session to ensure that the pressure is comfortable and effective.

There are several techniques used in shiatsu, including finger pressure, kneading, stretching, and rocking. These techniques can be combined and adapted to address specific areas of tension and promote relaxation. For example, kneading can be effective for releasing tight muscles in the back, while stretching can help to improve flexibility and range of motion.

Adapting pressure and technique in shiatsu can also be important for clients with specific health concerns. For example, clients with injuries or chronic pain may require a more gentle approach, while those with muscular tension may benefit from deeper pressure. It is important for the practitioner to have a thorough understanding of the client's health history and current condition in order to tailor the massage to their needs.

Another factor to consider when adapting pressure and technique in shiatsu is the client's age and physical condition. Elderly clients may require a lighter touch and more gentle stretches to avoid strain or discomfort, while athletes and active individuals may require deeper pressure to address tight muscles and promote recovery.

In addition to adjusting pressure and technique during the massage, it is also important for the practitioner to provide aftercare advice to the client. This may include stretches, exercises, or lifestyle changes to promote ongoing relaxation and healing. By working with the client to create a personalized aftercare plan, the practitioner can help to ensure that the benefits of shiatsu are maximized and maintained over time.

Chapter Sixteen

Shiatsu for Children and Pets

Shiatsu, an ancient Japanese healing practice, is known to provide various health benefits to adults. But did you know that it can also benefit children and even pets? Below we will explore the benefits of Shiatsu for children and pets and how it can be practiced safely.

Shiatsu is based on the principles of Traditional Chinese Medicine (TCM), which emphasize the flow of energy or qi (pronounced chee) through the body. This energy is believed to circulate through the body along specific pathways called meridians. The goal of Shiatsu is to balance the flow of energy through the meridians by applying pressure to specific points on the body.

For children, Shiatsu can help with various issues such as stress, anxiety, and even hyperactivity. It is believed that children's energy is more prone to becoming unbalanced due to their still-developing bodies and minds. Shiatsu can help to restore balance and promote relaxation in children.

One of the most important benefits of Shiatsu for children is that it is a non-invasive therapy that can be done without the need for medications. It is also safe and gentle, making it a good option for children who may be nervous about traditional therapies.

Shiatsu can also be practiced on pets. Pets are often an integral part of a family and providing them with Shiatsu can help them to relax and improve their overall well-being. Shiatsu can be used to address various issues in pets such as anxiety, muscle tension, and even digestive problems.

Shiatsu for pets is similar to that for humans in that it involves applying pressure to specific points on the body to balance the flow of energy. The pressure is applied using the fingers, palms, or elbows, depending on the size and sensitivity of the animal.

One important thing to note is that Shiatsu should only be practiced by those who are trained and qualified to do so. For children, it is important to seek out a practitioner who has experience working with children, as their bodies are still developing and may require a different approach.

When it comes to pets, it is important to work with a practitioner who has experience working with animals. Pets may react differently to Shiatsu than humans, so it is important to work with someone who is familiar with their behaviors and needs.

In addition to seeking out qualified practitioners, it is important to practice Shiatsu safely. When working with children, it is important to ensure that they are comfortable and relaxed. Practitioners should also be aware of any medical conditions or allergies the child may have.

When working with pets, it is important to work in a quiet and calm environment, as animals can be easily stressed. Practitioners should also be aware of any injuries or sensitivities the animal may have and adjust their technique accordingly.

Gentle techniques for young ones

Shiatsu is a Japanese bodywork therapy that involves applying pressure to specific points on the body. It is a gentle, non-invasive therapy that has been used for centuries to promote health and wellness. While Shiatsu is often associated with adult clients, it is also a suitable therapy for children and can even be used for pets. Below we will explore the gentle techniques used in Shiatsu for young ones.

Shiatsu for children is a gentle and effective therapy that can be used to promote physical and emotional well-being. Children can benefit from Shiatsu in many ways, including reducing stress, promoting relaxation, improving sleep, and boosting the immune system. Shiatsu can also help children who are suffering from conditions such as ADHD, anxiety, and depression.

One of the primary benefits of Shiatsu for children is its gentle nature. Unlike some other therapies, Shiatsu does not involve manipulation of the bones or joints. Instead, the therapist applies gentle pressure to specific points on the body. This makes Shiatsu a safe and non-invasive therapy for children.

When working with young clients, a Shiatsu therapist will typically use a lighter touch and will adapt their techniques to suit the child's age and developmental stage. For example, a therapist working with a young child may incorporate playful elements into the session, such as singing or storytelling, to help the child feel at ease. For older children, a therapist may use more specific techniques that target particular areas of the body.

There are several gentle techniques used in Shiatsu for children. One such technique is called the "holding technique." This technique involves placing the hands on the child's body and holding the pressure for several seconds. This technique can be used to promote relaxation and to release tension in the body.

Another technique commonly used in Shiatsu for children is the "brushing technique." This technique involves gently brushing the skin with the fingertips. This technique can be used to stimulate circulation and to help the child relax.

The "rocking technique" is another technique used in Shiatsu for children. This technique involves gently rocking the child's body back and forth. This can be a soothing and calming technique, particularly for young children.

Shiatsu can also be used for pets, particularly dogs and cats. Shiatsu for pets involves using gentle pressure on specific points on the body to promote relaxation and well-being. Shiatsu can be particularly beneficial for older pets who may be experiencing joint pain or mobility issues.

When working with pets, a Shiatsu therapist will typically use a light touch and will adapt their techniques to suit the animal's size and temperament. For example, a therapist working with a small dog may use techniques such as the "holding technique" or the "brushing technique," while a therapist working with a larger dog may use more specific techniques that target particular areas of the body.

Shiatsu for dogs and cats

Shiatsu, a Japanese massage therapy, can be beneficial not only for humans but also for their furry companions. Dogs and cats are prone to muscle tension, stress, and pain, just like humans, and Shiatsu can help alleviate their discomfort. Below we will explore the benefits of Shiatsu for pets, the techniques used, and the precautions to take.

Shiatsu is based on the principles of Traditional Chinese Medicine (TCM), which states that the body has a system of meridians or energy channels that are responsible for the proper functioning of organs and tissues. When these meridians become blocked or imbalanced, it can result in various ailments. Shiatsu aims to restore the balance of the body's energy flow by applying pressure to specific points on the meridians. The pressure applied is generally firm but gentle, and the techniques used are based on the principles of TCM.

Dogs and cats can benefit from Shiatsu in many ways. For instance, Shiatsu can help reduce muscle tension, improve circulation, boost the immune system, and reduce stress and anxiety. It can also help alleviate pain from arthritis or other joint problems. Shiatsu is a non-invasive therapy that can be used alone or in conjunction with other treatments.

The techniques used in Shiatsu for pets are similar to those used for humans. The therapist uses their fingers, thumbs, and palms to apply pressure to specific points on the pet's body. They may also use stretching and range-of-motion techniques to improve flexibility and mobility. However, the pressure applied is usually gentler than what is used for humans.

Before starting a Shiatsu session, it is essential to ensure that the pet is comfortable and relaxed. The therapist should approach the animal calmly and slowly, allowing them to sniff and become familiar with them. They should also be aware of the pet's body language and adjust their approach accordingly. If the pet seems uncomfortable or agitated, the session should be stopped.

It is also crucial to ensure that the pet is in good health before starting a Shiatsu session. If the pet has any underlying health conditions, it is best to consult with a veterinarian first. The therapist should also avoid areas of the body that are sore or inflamed and adjust their pressure accordingly.

Precautions and safety tips

Shiatsu, a form of bodywork that originated in Japan, can be a powerful tool for promoting relaxation, relieving tension, and supporting overall wellness. Like any form of manual therapy, however, there are certain precautions and safety tips to keep in mind when practicing or receiving shiatsu.

First and foremost, it is important to ensure that both the giver and receiver of shiatsu are comfortable and at ease. This means creating a safe and comfortable space in which to practice, with appropriate lighting, temperature, and other factors that contribute to relaxation and comfort.

In addition to creating a comfortable environment, it is important to ensure that both the giver and receiver are physically comfortable throughout the session. This may involve providing additional cushions or supports, adjusting the position of the body, or making other modifications to ensure that the client is not experiencing any pain or discomfort during the treatment.

Another important consideration when practicing shiatsu is the use of appropriate pressure and techniques. While shiatsu typically involves applying pressure to specific points on the body, it is important to be mindful of the amount of pressure being applied, as well as the techniques being used. For example, certain techniques may be more appropriate for certain individuals or conditions, while others may be contraindicated.

It is also important to be aware of any potential contraindications or precautions related to specific health conditions or medications. For example, shiatsu may not be appropriate for individuals with certain types of cancer, or for those who are taking certain medications that can affect blood pressure or other factors. It is always a good idea to consult with a healthcare professional before beginning any new form of bodywork, particularly if you have any underlying health conditions or concerns.

In addition to these general precautions and safety tips, there are also certain guidelines that can be followed to help ensure a safe and effective shiatsu session. For example, it is important to begin with a thorough assessment of the client's overall health and well-being, including any relevant medical history or current medications. This can help to identify any potential contraindications or concerns, and can also inform the selection of appropriate techniques and pressure levels.

Another important consideration when practicing shiatsu is the use of appropriate hygiene and sanitation practices. This may include using clean linens and towels, washing hands before and after the session, and disinfecting any equipment or surfaces that come into contact with the client's skin.

Finally, it is important to be aware of your own limitations as a shiatsu practitioner, and to seek out additional training or support as needed. This may involve continuing education courses, working with a mentor or supervisor, or consulting with other healthcare professionals as appropriate.

Chapter Seventeen

Advanced Shiatsu Techniques

Shiatsu is a Japanese healing technique that uses finger pressure to relieve tension and pain in the body. It is a form of bodywork that is based on the principles of Traditional Chinese Medicine (TCM) and the concept of energy flow in the body. Shiatsu is known for its ability to provide deep relaxation, reduce stress, and improve overall health and well-being. In addition to the basic techniques, there are also advanced Shiatsu techniques that can be used to address specific issues and conditions.

One of the advanced Shiatsu techniques is called "anma," which involves the use of fast, rhythmic movements to stimulate the flow of energy in the body. Anma can be used to relieve tension and pain, and to promote relaxation and overall health. Another technique is "stretching," which involves the use of stretching movements to release tension in the muscles and joints. This technique is particularly useful for people who suffer from tightness and stiffness in the body.

Another advanced Shiatsu technique is called "tsubo therapy," which involves the use of pressure on specific points on the body to stimulate the flow of energy and promote healing. Tsubo therapy is similar to acupressure, which is another healing technique that is based on the principles of TCM. Both Shiatsu and acupressure are believed to work by restoring the balance of energy in the body.

There are also advanced Shiatsu techniques that are designed to address specific conditions and issues. For example, Shiatsu can be used to relieve menstrual cramps, headaches, and digestive problems. It can also be used to promote fertility and relieve the symptoms of menopause. Shiatsu has also been found to be effective in treating chronic pain, such as back pain and arthritis.

One of the key principles of Shiatsu is that it is a holistic approach to healing that addresses the physical, emotional, and spiritual aspects of a person. This means that Shiatsu practitioners may also use other techniques, such as meditation, mindfulness, and visualization, to promote healing and balance in the body.

While advanced Shiatsu techniques can be effective in promoting healing and relieving specific conditions, it is important to remember that Shiatsu should not be used as a replacement for medical care. If you are experiencing a serious health condition or have concerns about your health, it is important to seek the advice of a qualified medical professional.

In addition to seeking medical care, there are also precautions and safety tips that should be followed when practicing Shiatsu. For example, Shiatsu should not be performed on areas of the body that are injured or inflamed. It is also important to communicate with your Shiatsu practitioner about any health concerns or issues that you may have, and to make sure that you are comfortable with the pressure and techniques that are being used.

Joint mobilization

Shiatsu is a form of Japanese massage that uses finger pressure and stretching to release tension and promote relaxation. One of the techniques used in Shiatsu is joint mobilization, which is a gentle yet effective way to help increase range of motion and reduce pain in the joints.

Joint mobilization involves moving the joint through its full range of motion, using gentle pressure and rhythmic movements. It is often used in conjunction with other Shiatsu techniques to help improve circulation, reduce muscle tension, and promote overall health and well-being.

One of the key benefits of joint mobilization is that it can help reduce pain and stiffness in the joints. This can be particularly helpful for people who suffer from conditions such as arthritis, which can cause joint pain and inflammation. By gently moving the joint through its full range of motion, joint mobilization can help improve joint function and reduce pain and stiffness.

In addition to reducing joint pain, joint mobilization can also help improve flexibility and range of motion. As we age, our joints can become stiff and less mobile, which can make it difficult to perform everyday tasks. By using gentle pressure and rhythmic movements to mobilize the joints, Shiatsu practitioners can help improve joint mobility and reduce the risk of injury.

Joint mobilization can be particularly helpful for athletes and people who engage in regular physical activity. By improving joint mobility, athletes can reduce their risk of injury and improve their performance. Joint mobilization can also help improve recovery time after a workout or competition, allowing athletes to get back to their training more quickly.

While joint mobilization is generally safe for most people, there are some precautions that should be taken. People with certain medical conditions, such as osteoporosis or joint hypermobility, may need to avoid joint mobilization or work with a Shiatsu practitioner who has experience working with these conditions. It is also important to communicate any discomfort or pain during a joint mobilization session, as this can be a sign that the technique is not appropriate for your individual needs.

Visceral manipulation

Visceral manipulation is a manual therapy technique that involves manipulating the internal organs in order to improve their function and mobility. This technique is often used in conjunction with Shiatsu and other forms of bodywork to address a wide range of physical and emotional issues.

The organs in our body are surrounded by connective tissue and held in place by ligaments and other structures. When this tissue becomes restricted or tight, it can limit the mobility of the organ, causing pain, discomfort, and other symptoms. Visceral manipulation works by using gentle pressure and stretching techniques to release these restrictions and improve the mobility and function of the organs.

Visceral manipulation is based on the principle that the body is interconnected and that the health of one organ or system can affect the health of the entire body. For example, restrictions in the liver can cause problems with digestion, while restrictions in the lungs can affect breathing and respiratory function.

During a visceral manipulation session, the practitioner will use their hands to gently manipulate the organs and surrounding tissue, assessing for areas of tension and restriction. The practitioner will then use various techniques to release the tension and improve the mobility of the organ.

There are many benefits to visceral manipulation, including improved organ function, reduced pain and discomfort, improved digestion and elimination, improved breathing, and improved immune function. This technique can also help to reduce stress and promote relaxation, which can have a positive impact on overall health and wellbeing.

In addition to Shiatsu, visceral manipulation is often used in conjunction with other forms of bodywork and manual therapy, such as massage, osteopathy, and chiropractic. It can also be used as part of a comprehensive treatment plan for a wide range of health conditions, including digestive issues, respiratory problems, and chronic pain.

It is important to note that visceral manipulation should only be performed by a trained and licensed practitioner, as the technique involves working with internal organs and can pose certain risks if not performed correctly. Additionally, certain medical conditions may not be appropriate for visceral manipulation, and it is important to consult with a healthcare professional before undergoing this type of therapy.

Craniosacral therapy

Craniosacral therapy is a gentle yet powerful bodywork technique that works with the craniosacral system, which consists of the membranes and cerebrospinal fluid that surround and protect the brain and spinal cord. This therapy aims to release tensions and restrictions in the craniosacral system to improve the body's overall health and well-being.

Craniosacral therapy is often used to treat a wide range of conditions, including headaches, chronic pain, anxiety, depression, and stress-related disorders. It is also used to improve the immune system, enhance neurological function, and promote deep relaxation.

During a craniosacral therapy session, the practitioner will use light touch and gentle pressure to detect and release areas of tension or restriction in the craniosacral system. The therapist will typically start by evaluating the client's body for signs of tension or imbalance, such as asymmetry or restricted movement.

Once the areas of tension have been identified, the therapist will use gentle touch and pressure to help release these restrictions. This can involve light massage, stretching, or gentle manipulation of the bones of the skull, spine, and pelvis.

One of the key principles of craniosacral therapy is that the body has an inherent ability to heal itself. By working with the craniosacral system, the therapist can help to activate this natural healing process and promote optimal health and well-being.

Research has shown that craniosacral therapy can be effective in reducing pain, anxiety, and depression, and improving sleep quality and overall quality of life. It has also been shown to be effective in treating conditions such as migraines, fibromyalgia, and chronic fatigue syndrome.

While craniosacral therapy is generally considered safe, it is important to seek out a qualified practitioner who has received adequate training and certification. It is also important to discuss any health conditions or concerns with your practitioner before beginning treatment.

In addition to craniosacral therapy, there are several other techniques that can be used to promote overall health and well-being. Shiatsu, for example, is a Japanese form of bodywork that uses finger pressure to stimulate the body's natural healing processes.

Like craniosacral therapy, shiatsu works with the body's energy meridians to promote balance and harmony throughout the body. It can be effective in treating a wide range of conditions, including musculoskeletal pain, stress-related disorders, and digestive issues.

Another technique that can be used to promote overall health and well-being is acupuncture. This traditional Chinese medicine technique involves the insertion of thin needles into specific points on the body to promote healing and balance.

Acupuncture has been shown to be effective in treating a wide range of conditions, including pain, anxiety, and depression, and is often used in conjunction with other therapies such as massage and herbal medicine.

When seeking out craniosacral therapy or any other bodywork technique, it is important to find a qualified practitioner who has received adequate training and certification. It is also important to discuss any health concerns or conditions with your practitioner before beginning treatment. By working with a qualified practitioner and taking an active role in your own health and wellness, you can help to promote optimal health and well-being.

Chapter Eighteen

Shiatsu and Spirituality

Shiatsu is a form of bodywork that originated in Japan and is based on the principles of Traditional Chinese Medicine (TCM). It involves the application of pressure and stretching techniques to specific points on the body, with the aim of promoting relaxation, improving circulation, and balancing the flow of energy (qi) throughout the body. While Shiatsu is often seen as a physical therapy, it can also have spiritual dimensions, and many practitioners and recipients of Shiatsu report experiencing a sense of deep relaxation, connection, and even spiritual transformation during sessions.

In TCM, the human body is seen as a complex system of interrelated parts, including physical, mental, emotional, and spiritual components. According to this worldview, health and wellbeing depend on the balance and harmonious flow of qi, the vital energy that animates all living beings. Shiatsu is one of the modalities that aims to restore this balance by working with the body's energy channels (meridians) and acupressure points, which are believed to correspond to different organs, emotions, and aspects of the self.

While Shiatsu does not have a specific spiritual tradition associated with it, it can be seen as part of a broader movement towards integrating mind-body-spirit approaches to health and wellbeing. Many people who practice or receive Shiatsu report feeling a sense of connection, peace, and even transcendence during sessions, which can be interpreted as spiritual experiences. Some practitioners also incorporate mindfulness, visualization, and other spiritual practices into their Shiatsu sessions, with the aim of promoting relaxation, self-awareness, and connection to a higher power.

One of the ways in which Shiatsu can have spiritual dimensions is through the use of intention and presence. Shiatsu practitioners are trained to approach their work with a deep sense of presence, compassion, and non-judgment, which can create a safe and supportive space for clients to relax and release physical and emotional tension. The intention of the practitioner is also an important aspect of Shiatsu, as it can help to focus the energy and promote healing. Some practitioners use visualization or other techniques to set a positive intention for each session, such as promoting relaxation, releasing pain, or cultivating inner peace.

Another way in which Shiatsu can have spiritual dimensions is through the use of symbols and metaphors. In TCM, each meridian and acupressure point is associated with a specific organ, emotion, or aspect of the self. For example, the liver meridian is said to be associated with anger and frustration, while the heart meridian is associated with love and joy. By working with these points and meridians, Shiatsu practitioners can help clients to release emotional blockages and access deeper levels of awareness and understanding. Some practitioners also use symbols or metaphors to help clients to connect with their inner selves and promote healing. For example, a practitioner might use the image of a river flowing smoothly to help a client release emotional tension and promote the flow of qi.

Finally, Shiatsu can have spiritual dimensions through the promotion of self-awareness and self-care. Many people who receive Shiatsu report feeling more connected to their bodies, emotions, and inner selves, which can lead to greater self-awareness and a deeper sense of purpose. Some practitioners also encourage clients to practice self-care techniques at home, such as meditation, visualization, or gentle movement, which can promote spiritual growth and wellbeing.

The mind-body connection

The mind and body are intricately connected, and it is widely accepted that our mental and emotional states can have a significant impact on our physical health. This connection has been observed and studied for centuries by Eastern cultures, including those that practice Shiatsu.

Shiatsu is a form of Japanese massage therapy that uses finger pressure on specific points of the body to relieve tension and pain. It is based on the principles of Traditional Chinese Medicine (TCM), which views the body as an interconnected system of energy channels, or meridians. Shiatsu aims to balance the flow of energy, or qi, throughout the body to promote overall health and well-being.

One of the unique aspects of Shiatsu is its focus on the mind-body connection. Practitioners believe that emotions and stress can cause blockages in the flow of energy, leading to physical tension and pain. Therefore, Shiatsu techniques are designed not only to address physical symptoms but also to promote emotional and mental relaxation and balance.

In Shiatsu, the mind and body are seen as inseparable. The techniques used are designed to work on both physical and emotional levels simultaneously, helping to promote a sense of wholeness and harmony. By working with the body's energy channels, Shiatsu aims to promote deep relaxation, reduce stress and anxiety, and improve overall mental and emotional well-being.

There are several ways in which Shiatsu can help promote the mind-body connection. First, Shiatsu helps to release physical tension and pain, which can have a direct impact on our emotional and mental states. When we experience physical pain, it can be difficult to focus, stay positive, or feel emotionally balanced. By releasing physical tension, Shiatsu can help promote mental clarity, emotional stability, and a sense of calm.

Secondly, Shiatsu helps to promote relaxation and reduce stress. When we experience stress, our bodies respond with physical symptoms, such as tension, headaches, and digestive problems. Shiatsu techniques, such as gentle stretching and pressure on specific points, help to activate the parasympathetic nervous system, which is responsible for promoting relaxation and reducing stress.

Thirdly, Shiatsu can help to improve our body awareness and promote mindfulness. By focusing on specific points of the body and being present in the moment, Shiatsu can help us become more aware of our physical sensations and promote mindfulness. This can help us become more in tune with our bodies and emotions, which can promote overall well-being and happiness.

Cultivating mindfulness and presence

Cultivating mindfulness and presence is an essential aspect of practicing Shiatsu. Shiatsu is a form of Japanese bodywork that involves applying pressure to specific points on the body to help balance the body's energy and promote healing. The practice of Shiatsu requires practitioners to be fully present and aware of their own body, mind, and emotions as well as those of their clients.

Mindfulness is the practice of being present and fully engaged in the moment, without judgment or distraction. It involves paying attention to physical sensations, emotions, and thoughts as they arise, and learning to observe them without getting caught up in them. Mindfulness is essential for Shiatsu practitioners because it allows them to be fully present with their clients, and to tune in to their clients' needs and responses.

One way to cultivate mindfulness and presence in Shiatsu is through meditation. Meditation is a practice of training the mind to be calm and focused. It involves sitting quietly, focusing on the breath, and letting go of distracting thoughts and emotions. Meditation can help Shiatsu practitioners to develop a greater awareness of their own body, mind, and emotions, which can help them to be more present and attentive with their clients.

Another way to cultivate mindfulness and presence in Shiatsu is through the practice of Qi Gong. Qi Gong is a Chinese practice of gentle movements, breathing exercises, and meditation that promotes health and well-being. Qi Gong can help Shiatsu practitioners to develop a greater awareness of their own energy, and to learn how to sense and work with the energy of their clients.

In addition to meditation and Qi Gong, there are other practices that can help Shiatsu practitioners to cultivate mindfulness and presence. These include yoga, Tai Chi, and other forms of bodywork. These practices can help to develop greater body awareness, and can help to release tension and stress, which can interfere with a practitioner's ability to be fully present with their clients.

Cultivating mindfulness and presence is essential for effective Shiatsu practice, as it helps practitioners to be fully present with their clients, and to tune in to their clients' needs and responses. By developing greater awareness of their own body, mind, and emotions, Shiatsu practitioners can develop greater sensitivity and intuition, which can help them to work more effectively with their clients' energy.

Exploring energy work and chakras

Exploring Energy Work and Chakras in Shiatsu

Shiatsu is a form of Japanese bodywork that involves the application of pressure on specific points of the body to balance the body's energy or "Ki." This energy flows through the body's energy channels, also known as meridians, and is associated with the various internal organs and systems. In Shiatsu, the practitioner works to stimulate or soothe these points to promote overall health and wellbeing.

One of the central concepts in Shiatsu is the idea of energy centers, also known as chakras, which are believed to be located along the body's mid-line. The chakras are associated with different emotional and physical aspects of our being and are thought to influence our overall health and wellbeing.

In Shiatsu, each chakra is associated with a specific meridian and internal organ system. By working on the chakras, a Shiatsu practitioner can help to balance the body's energy and promote overall health and wellbeing.

Let's take a closer look at the seven chakras and their associated meridians and organs:

1. Root Chakra: This chakra is located at the base of the spine and is associated with the large intestine meridian and the adrenal gland. It is associated with grounding and stability, and is thought to influence our sense of security and basic survival needs.

2. Sacral Chakra: This chakra is located in the lower abdomen and is associated with the kidney meridian and the reproductive organs. It is associated with creativity and sexuality, and is thought to influence our sense of pleasure and emotional balance.

3. Solar Plexus Chakra: This chakra is located in the upper abdomen and is associated with the stomach meridian and the pancreas. It is associated with personal power and confidence, and is thought to influence our sense of self-worth and identity.

4. Heart Chakra: This chakra is located in the center of the chest and is associated with the heart meridian and the thymus gland. It is associated with love and compassion, and is thought to influence our ability to connect with others and experience empathy.

5. Throat Chakra: This chakra is located in the throat and is associated with the lung meridian and the thyroid gland. It is associated with communication and self-expression, and is thought to influence our ability to speak our truth and express ourselves authentically.

6. Third Eye Chakra: This chakra is located in the center of the forehead and is associated with the bladder meridian and the pituitary gland. It is associated with intuition and insight, and is thought to influence our ability to connect with our inner wisdom and make decisions.

7. Crown Chakra: This chakra is located at the top of the head and is associated with the governing vessel meridian and the pineal gland. It is associated with spirituality and connection to the divine, and is thought to influence our sense of purpose and connection to something greater than ourselves.

In Shiatsu, the practitioner may use a combination of pressure, stretching, and joint manipulation techniques to stimulate or soothe the meridians and chakras as needed. This may involve applying pressure to specific points on the body, or working with the body's energy field to promote balance and harmony.

While the concept of chakras may be unfamiliar to those new to Shiatsu, it is important to note that the practice of Shiatsu is rooted in a holistic understanding of the body and its interconnected systems. By working with the body's energy flow and promoting balance and harmony, Shiatsu can be a powerful tool for promoting overall health and wellbeing.

In addition to Shiatsu, there are many other energy-based modalities that work with the body's chakras and energy field, including Reiki,

Chapter Nineteen

Case Studies and Success Stories

Shiatsu is a Japanese form of massage therapy that uses finger pressure on specific areas of the body to promote healing and relaxation. It has been found to be effective in treating a wide range of physical and emotional conditions, and many people have reported success in improving their health and well-being through regular Shiatsu sessions. Below we will explore some case studies and success stories that demonstrate the effectiveness of Shiatsu in various contexts.

One common use of Shiatsu is for the treatment of chronic pain. In a case study published in the International Journal of Therapeutic Massage and Bodywork, a 46-year-old woman with chronic lower back pain received eight weekly Shiatsu sessions. By the end of the treatment period, the woman reported a significant decrease in pain intensity and improved quality of life. She also reported feeling more relaxed and less stressed overall.

Another study, published in the Journal of Bodywork and Movement Therapies, explored the use of Shiatsu in reducing symptoms of depression and anxiety. In the study, participants received six weekly Shiatsu sessions, and their symptoms were assessed before and after the treatment period. The researchers found that Shiatsu was effective in reducing symptoms of both depression and anxiety, and that these improvements were sustained over time.

Shiatsu has also been found to be effective in treating various conditions related to women's health. In a study published in the Journal of Alternative and Complementary Medicine, women with menstrual pain received five weekly Shiatsu treatments. The researchers found that Shiatsu was effective in reducing both the intensity and duration of menstrual pain, as well as improving overall quality of life.

Shiatsu has also been used successfully in the treatment of cancer patients. In a study published in the Journal of Complementary and Integrative Medicine, breast cancer patients receiving chemotherapy received six weekly Shiatsu treatments. The patients reported significant improvements in quality of life, including reduced fatigue, improved sleep, and decreased nausea and vomiting.

Success stories with Shiatsu are not limited to physical conditions. In a case study published in the Journal of Bodywork and Movement Therapies, a 24-year-old woman with severe social anxiety received six weekly Shiatsu sessions. By the end of the treatment period, the woman reported significant reductions in anxiety symptoms and improved quality of life. She also reported feeling more confident and socially connected.

Another case study, published in the Journal of Holistic Nursing, explored the use of Shiatsu in treating insomnia in a 40-year-old woman. The woman received five weekly Shiatsu sessions, and reported significant improvements in sleep quality and a decrease in sleep medication usage.

These case studies and success stories demonstrate the wide-ranging benefits of Shiatsu. While more research is needed to fully understand the mechanisms by which Shiatsu works, there is a growing body of evidence to support its effectiveness in treating various physical and emotional conditions. If you are interested in exploring Shiatsu for yourself, it is important to find a qualified practitioner who can provide personalized treatment based on your individual needs and goals.

Real-life examples of healing

Shiatsu is a Japanese massage therapy that focuses on applying pressure to specific points on the body to relieve tension and promote overall health and wellness. It is based on the principles of traditional Chinese medicine and emphasizes the balance of energy in the body. Although Shiatsu is not a substitute for medical treatment, it can be used as a complementary therapy to help manage a variety of physical and emotional conditions. Here are some real-life examples of how Shiatsu has helped individuals on their path to healing.

Chronic Pain Management

One common condition that Shiatsu can help manage is chronic pain. A case study published in the Journal of Integrative Medicine reported that a 72-year-old woman with chronic back pain experienced significant pain relief after receiving Shiatsu treatments twice a week for four weeks. The study also noted that the woman's quality of life improved, and she was able to reduce her use of pain medication.

Another study published in the Journal of Traditional Chinese Medicine described a 45-year-old woman with chronic shoulder pain who received Shiatsu treatments twice a week for four weeks. The study reported that the woman experienced a significant reduction in pain intensity and an improvement in her range of motion.

Anxiety and Depression

Shiatsu can also help manage symptoms of anxiety and depression. A study published in the Journal of Alternative and Complementary Medicine reported that 12 weeks of weekly Shiatsu treatments led to significant improvements in anxiety, depression, and quality of life among participants with anxiety disorders. Another study published in the Journal of Psychiatric Research found that 12 weeks of biweekly Shiatsu treatments reduced depression and anxiety symptoms in patients with major depressive disorder.

Pregnancy and Postpartum Support

Shiatsu can also be beneficial during pregnancy and postpartum. A case study published in the Journal of Bodywork and Movement Therapies described a 32-year-old woman who received Shiatsu treatments during her pregnancy to manage nausea, insomnia, and low back pain. The study reported that the woman experienced significant improvements in all of these symptoms.

Another case study published in the same journal described a 35-year-old woman who received Shiatsu treatments postpartum to manage fatigue, anxiety, and difficulty sleeping. The study reported that the woman experienced significant improvements in all of these symptoms and was able to discontinue the use of sleep medication.

Overall Health and Wellness

Shiatsu can also be used as a preventative measure to promote overall health and wellness. A study published in the Journal of Alternative and Complementary Medicine found that weekly Shiatsu treatments for eight weeks led to significant improvements in sleep quality and immune function among healthy adults.

Another study published in the Journal of Bodywork and Movement Therapies found that biweekly Shiatsu treatments for 12 weeks led to significant improvements in perceived stress and quality of life among university students.

Testimonials from practitioners

Shiatsu, a traditional Japanese healing art, has been gaining popularity around the world due to its many benefits. Practitioners of this technique have been sharing their experiences and testimonials to spread awareness about the healing powers of Shiatsu.

Shiatsu is a form of massage that uses finger pressure and other techniques to stimulate the body's energy flow. It is based on the principles of Traditional Chinese Medicine and aims to balance the body's energy to promote healing and wellness.

One of the main benefits of Shiatsu is its ability to reduce stress and promote relaxation. Many practitioners have reported that their clients feel more relaxed and less stressed after a Shiatsu session. This is because Shiatsu stimulates the parasympathetic nervous system, which helps the body relax and reduce stress.

Shiatsu has also been known to relieve pain and tension in the body. Practitioners have shared testimonials of clients experiencing relief from headaches, back pain, and other types of chronic pain after Shiatsu sessions. This is because Shiatsu helps improve circulation, reduce inflammation, and release tension in the muscles.

In addition to physical benefits, Shiatsu has also been known to improve mental and emotional well-being. Practitioners have reported that clients feel more centered and grounded after a Shiatsu session. This is because Shiatsu helps balance the body's energy, which can help reduce anxiety, depression, and other mental health issues.

Many practitioners have also shared success stories of clients with specific conditions finding relief through Shiatsu. For example, one practitioner shared the story of a client with fibromyalgia who had been struggling with chronic pain for years. After regular Shiatsu sessions, the client reported significant improvements in pain and mobility.

Another practitioner shared a story of a client with digestive issues who had been suffering from chronic constipation for years. After just a few Shiatsu sessions, the client reported improved digestion and regular bowel movements.

Practitioners have also shared testimonials of their own personal experiences with Shiatsu. Many have reported that practicing Shiatsu regularly has helped them become more centered, grounded, and present in their daily lives.

In addition to the testimonials of practitioners and clients, there is also scientific research supporting the benefits of Shiatsu. Studies have shown that Shiatsu can help reduce anxiety, depression, and other mental health issues, as well as improve physical symptoms such as pain and mobility.

Lessons learned and insights gained

Shiatsu is an ancient Japanese healing practice that involves the application of pressure to specific points on the body to promote relaxation, relieve stress, and alleviate various health conditions. Over the years, practitioners and clients alike have reported numerous benefits from receiving Shiatsu treatments. Below we will explore some of the lessons learned and insights gained from the practice of Shiatsu.

One of the most significant insights gained from Shiatsu is the importance of relaxation and stress reduction for overall health and wellbeing. In today's fast-paced world, stress is an all too common experience that can lead to a host of physical and mental health problems. Through the practice of Shiatsu, individuals can learn to release tension and let go of stress, leading to improved sleep, increased energy, and a greater sense of calm.

Another important lesson learned through Shiatsu is the power of touch in promoting healing and wellness. Many people today are disconnected from their bodies and their sense of touch, which can lead to feelings of isolation and disconnection. Through the practice of Shiatsu, individuals can learn to reconnect with their bodies and become more aware of their physical sensations. This heightened sense of awareness can lead to improved self-care practices and a greater appreciation for the body's ability to heal itself.

Shiatsu can also provide insights into the interconnectedness of the body, mind, and spirit. Many clients report feeling a sense of inner peace and emotional release during Shiatsu sessions. This can be attributed to the fact that Shiatsu stimulates the body's natural healing processes and can help to release blocked energy and emotions. By addressing both physical and emotional issues, Shiatsu can provide a holistic approach to healing that addresses the root causes of many health problems.

Another insight gained from Shiatsu is the importance of self-care and personal responsibility for one's health. Through regular Shiatsu sessions, clients can become more attuned to their bodies and learn to recognize when something is not right. They can also learn self-massage techniques and other self-care practices to maintain their health and wellbeing between sessions. This empowerment can lead to improved self-esteem and a greater sense of control over one's health.

Shiatsu can also provide lessons on the importance of individualized treatment. Unlike Western medicine, which often takes a one-size-fits-all approach to treatment, Shiatsu recognizes that each individual is unique and requires a personalized approach. Practitioners will take into account a client's physical and emotional needs, as well as their overall health and lifestyle, to create a treatment plan that is tailored to their specific needs. This personalized approach can lead to more effective and long-lasting results.

Finally, Shiatsu can provide insights into the power of human connection. Many people today feel disconnected from others and long for a sense of community and connection. Through the practice of Shiatsu, individuals can experience a sense of connection and intimacy with their practitioner, which can lead to a greater sense of belonging and wellbeing. Shiatsu also provides an opportunity for individuals to connect with their own bodies and their sense of self, leading to greater self-awareness and a deeper understanding of one's place in the world.

9781776968183
SD - #0055 - 140926 - C0 - 229/152/8 - PB - 9781776968183 - Matt Lamination